# Off Grid Survival Projects Bible

## How to Master Skills in Nature

Robin J. Snider

Copyright © 2024 Robin J. Snider

Tutti i diritti riservati.

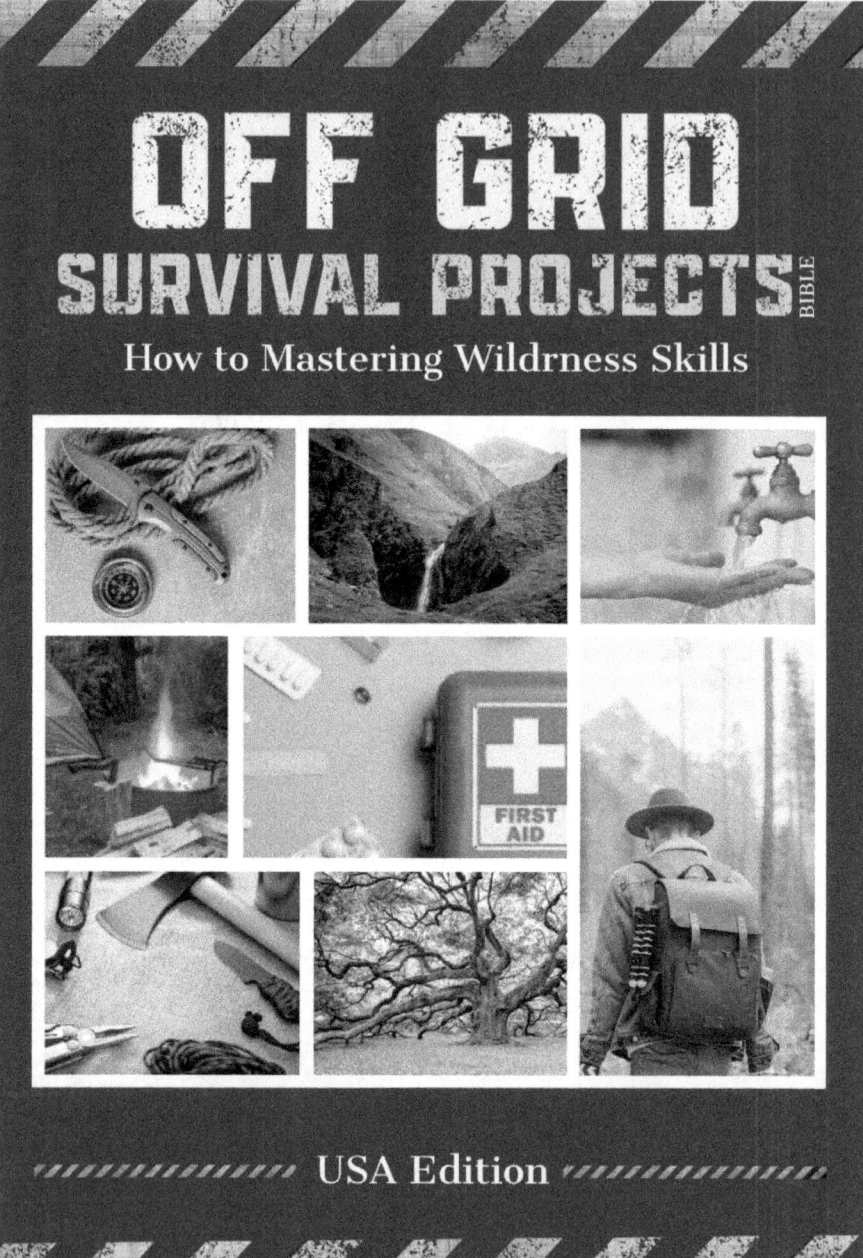

# Indice

Survival Mindset --------------------------------------------- 7
Introduction: Surviving off the grid ----------------------- 10
Purpose of the book --------------------------------------- 13
Importance of off-grid living ----------------------------- 13
Topic Overview. ------------------------------------------- 14
**Chapter 1.** ------------------------------------------------- **16**
**Introduction to the basics of off-grid living** ----------- **16**
Definition of off-grid living ------------------------------ 16
Benefits and challenges ----------------------------------- 18
**hapter 2.** -------------------------------------------------- **21**
**Water Resources** ----------------------------------------- **21**
Water Sources -------------------------------------------- 25
Collection of Rainwater ---------------------------------- 28
Construction of wells ------------------------------------ 28
Use of natural watercourses ------------------------------ 28
Water Treatment ----------------------------------------- 29
Filtrfation Methods -------------------------------------- 29
Solar Alembics ------------------------------------------- 29
Chemical treatment -------------------------------------- 30
Water storage and conservation -------------------------- 30
Sistema completo di raccolta e distribuzione ------------ 33
**Chapter 3.** ------------------------------------------------- **34**
**Food Sustainability** -------------------------------------- **34**
Food production ----------------------------------------- 34
Permaculture and sustainable agriculture ---------------- 38
Gardening in small spaces ------------------------------- 40
Growing fruit trees -------------------------------------- 41
Food supply --------------------------------------------- 43
Permaculture and Sustainable Agriculture --------------- 46

Gardening in Small Spaces ------------------------------------47

Urban gardens: ---------------------------------------------48

Small green areas used for growing vegetables and flowers --------------------------------------------------------48

Growing fruit trees ----------------------------------------48

Examples of Permaculture and Sustainable Agriculture--49

Procuring Food ---------------------------------------------50

Fisheries and aquaculture ---------------------------------51

How to store food ------------------------------------------53

**Chapter 4. -------------------------------------------------54**

**Construction of shelters -----------------------------------54**

Planning the shelter---------------------------------------54

Planning the Shelter --------------------------------------61

Choice of Location-----------------------------------------61

Example 1: Wooden shelter --------------------------------64

Example 2: Shelter in Earth and Straw --------------------65

**Capitolo 5.-------------------------------------------------67**

**Energia Rinnovabile----------------------------------------67**

Overview of Renewable Energy Options ------------------67

Solar --------------------------------------------------------68

Hydroelectric ----------------------------------------------73

Installazione di sistemi energetici -------------------------73

Micro-Hydro Systems --------------------------------------74

Energy management and maintenance ------------------74

**Chapter 6. -------------------------------------------------75**

**Emergency preparedness -----------------------------------75**

First aid ----------------------------------------------------75

Treatment of common wounds -----------------------------76

Preparazione di un kit di pronto soccorso-----------------77

Planning for natural disasters -----------------------------81

Evacuation strategies ------------------------------------ 82
Essential concepts for an evacuation plan ---------------- 83
Temporary shelters --------------------------------------- 86
Disaster response programme ------------------------------ 87

## Chapter 7.  ---------------------------------------------- 91
## Survival skills ----------------------------------------- 91

Light the fire ------------------------------------------- 91
Traditional and modern methods --------------------------- 91
Fuel storage --------------------------------------------- 92
Natural navigation techniques ---------------------------- 93
Craft techniques ----------------------------------------- 93
Wood and stone processing -------------------------------- 93
Manufacture of tools and weapons ------------------------- 94
Creation of clothing and accessories --------------------- 98

## Chapter 8. ---------------------------------------------- 102
## Living in harmony with nature -------------------------- 102

Conservation of natural resources ----------------------- 103
Education and Knowledge Sharing ------------------------- 103
Conclusion ---------------------------------------------- 105
Key Points Summary -------------------------------------- 105
Inspiration for off-grid life --------------------------- 106
Resources and suppliers --------------------------------- 107
Glossary of technical terms ----------------------------- 108

© Copyright 2024 by Robin J. Snider - Tutti i diritti riservati.

The following book is reproduced with the aim of providing the most accurate and reliable information possible. However, the purchase of this book may be taken as an agreement that both the publisher and the author of this book are in no way experts on the topics covered and that any recommendations or suggestions made here are for entertainment purposes only. Professional advice should be sought before taking any action recommended here. This statement is deemed correct and valid by both the American Bar Association and the Committee of Publishers Association and is legally binding throughout the United States. In addition, the transmission, duplication or reproduction of any of the following works, including specific information, will be considered an illegal act, regardless of whether it is done in electronic or printed form. This extends to the creation of a secondary or tertiary copy of the work or a recorded copy and is permitted only with the express written consent of the Publisher. All additional rights are reserved. The information contained in the following pages is generally considered a true and accurate account of the facts and, as such, any carelessness, use or misuse of such information by the reader will render any resulting action solely the responsibility of the reader. The publisher or the original author of this work can in no way be held responsible for any inconvenience or damage that may result from the use of the information described herein. Furthermore, the information contained in the following pages is intended for informational purposes only and should be considered universal. By their nature, they are presented without any guarantee of prolonged validity or intermediate quality. The trademarks cited are made without written consent and can in no way be considered an endorsement by the trademark owner.

**Survival Mindset**

In times of extreme adversity, it is often said that mindset is everything. This is especially true when it comes to the concept of survival mindset. Survival mindset is the mental strength and determination to overcome challenges and persevere in the face of danger or difficulty. It is the ability to adapt to unforeseen circumstances, make quick decisions and act to ensure one's survival. In this essay we will explore the importance of a survival mindset and how to cultivate it to increase our chances of survival in various situations.

One of the key aspects of a survival mindset is the ability to remain calm and focused under pressure. In survival situations, panic can be deadly, as it leads to making irrational decisions and ultimately putting one's life at risk. By keeping a clear mind and assessing the situation with a rational mindset, one can better evaluate options and take the necessary steps to ensure one's safety and well-being.

Another important component of survival mindset is adaptability. In a crisis situation, things can change quickly and unexpectedly. Those with a survival mindset are able to adapt quickly to changing circumstances, adjusting their plans and tactics as needed to increase their chances of survival. This flexibility and willingness to think independently are invaluable when facing unpredictable and dangerous situations.

Preparation is another crucial aspect of survival mindset. Those who are prepared are more likely to survive in emergency situations because they have the tools, skills and knowledge needed to effectively manage a crisis. This includes having a well-stocked emergency kit, knowing basic survival skills such as building a shelter or starting a fire, and having a plan in place for various scenarios. With preparedness, people can act quickly and decisively when faced with a life-threatening situation.

Resilience is also a key characteristic of survival mindset. Resilient people are able to recover from setbacks and difficulties by maintaining a strong spirit and determination to survive regardless of the odds. This mental toughness allows them to endure physical and emotional challenges, overcoming difficulties and coming out stronger on the other side. Without resilience, it is difficult to persevere in the face of adversity and overcome obstacles to survival.

Another important aspect of survival mindset is resourcefulness. In desperate situations, resources may be scarce, which requires individuals to think creatively and make the most of what they have. Resource aptitude involves the use of ingenuity and problem-solving skills to find solutions to challenges and make the best use of available resources. Those with a survival mindset are able to adapt and improvise to meet their basic needs and increase their chances of survival.

Survival mindset implies a relentless will to survive. This unwavering determination drives individuals to keep fighting for their lives, even when the odds seem insurmountable. This will to survive is often what separates those who die in life-threatening situations from those who manage to survive against all odds. By embodying a strong sense of purpose and a refusal to give up, individuals with a survival mindset can overcome even the most dire circumstances and emerge victorious in the end.

By cultivating mental strength, adaptability, preparedness, resilience, resourcefulness and a relentless will to survive, individuals can better cope with crises and emerge unscathed. By developing a survival mindset, not only can we increase our chances of survival in emergencies, but we can also build resilience and strength that can serve us in all areas of life.

## Introduction: Surviving off the grid

Living off the grid has become an increasingly popular lifestyle choice for many people seeking to simplify, reduce their environmental impact and become more self-sufficient. For those who want to embark on this journey, the "Off Grid Survival Bible" is an indispensable guide. This comprehensive handbook provides practical advice, essential tools and valuable tips for thriving in a self-sufficient, off-grid lifestyle.

One of the key aspects of off-grid living is ensuring access to clean water. The "Off-Grid Survival Bible" offers detailed information on how to collect, store and purify water from natural sources such as rainwater, streams and wells. The book also provides guidance on how to build water collection systems, water filters and other methods to ensure a safe and reliable water supply.

In addition to water, food is another essential element for off-grid survival. The "Off Grid Survival Bible" contains valuable information on growing your own food, raising livestock and foraging wild foods. The book details techniques for planting and growing crops, preserving food through canning and drying, and creating homemade fertilizers and pesticides.

Energy is another crucial aspect of off-grid living, and "Off-Grid Survival Bible" offers a wealth of information on energy generation and storage. From solar panels to wind turbines, small-scale hydropower systems to biomass generators, the book covers a wide range of renewable energy options. It also provides guidance on how to build energy-efficient homes, reduce energy consumption and live comfortably without being connected to the grid.

In addition to practical advice on water, food and energy, "Off Grid Survival Bible" also addresses essential skills for thriving in a self-sufficient lifestyle. The book covers topics such as wilderness survival, first aid, building a fire, shelter construction and navigation. It also includes tips on collecting medicinal plants, preparing herbal remedies and dealing with emergencies and natural disasters.

One of the biggest challenges of living off the grid is maintaining communication and contact with the outside world. The "Off-Grid Survival Bible" provides guidance on setting up communication systems such as two-way radios, satellite phones and Internet access. The book also offers advice on how to maintain personal relationships, stay informed about current events, and manage finances without traditional banking services.

Living off the grid can present unique challenges and obstacles, and "The Off-Grid Survival Bible" addresses these issues with practical solutions and expert advice. Whether it's extreme weather, wild animals or medical emergencies, the book provides strategies for staying safe and maintaining a healthy, sustainable lifestyle. It also offers tips for building resilient communities, forging partnerships with like-minded people, and creating a support network for mutual aid and assistance.

Packed with practical advice, essential tools and valuable tips, this comprehensive handbook provides all the information you need to thrive in a sustainable, independent lifestyle. Whether you are an experienced homesteader or new to off-grid living, this book is sure to become an indispensable guide and companion on your journey to self-sufficiency.

## Purpose of the book

The main purpose of "Off Grid Survival Bible" is to provide a comprehensive and practical guide for those who wish to live self-sufficiently, regardless of modern infrastructure. This book is designed for anyone who wants to prepare for emergencies, reduce their ecological footprint, or simply live a simpler life connected to nature. The guide offers detailed instructions, practical tips, and proven techniques for meeting the challenges of off-grid living, promoting greater awareness and self-sufficiency.

## Importance of off-grid living

Off-grid living is becoming increasingly important in a world characterized by climatic, economic, and social uncertainties. Independence from power grids not only provides security in case of natural emergencies or blackouts, but also promotes a more sustainable and environmentally friendly lifestyle. Off-grid living makes it possible to reduce dependence on fossil resources and adopt renewable energy, contributing to the fight against climate change. In addition, the development of survival skills and personal resilience can improve quality of life, promoting better health and overall well-being.

## Topic Overview.

The "Off-Grid Survival Bible" covers a wide range of topics critical to those who wish to live off-grid. It begins with the basics of self-sufficient living, exploring the benefits and challenges of this lifestyle and the mindset needed to deal with it successfully. The book then delves into water resources, explaining how to find, purify and conserve water, an essential element for survival.

A chapter on food sustainability follows, detailing food production, procurement and storage. It then moves on to shelter construction, offering instructions on how to design and build houses using natural and renewable materials. Renewable energy is another key topic, with a focus on solar, wind and hydropower.

Emergency preparedness, survival skills and the importance of living in harmony with nature are other crucial topics covered in the book. Each chapter is designed to provide practical and easily applicable knowledge so that readers can face the challenges of off-grid living with confidence.

The chapter on emergency preparedness explores how to deal with critical situations such as natural disasters, accidents and threats to personal safety, providing detailed instruction on first aid, self-defense and evacuation strategies. Survival skills include fire-starting techniques, navigation without modern tools, and crafts to create necessary tools and clothing.

Living in harmony with nature is fundamental to sustainable off-grid living. This chapter discusses the principles of environmental sustainability, conservation of natural resources and the importance of educating and sharing knowledge with the community. The "Off-Grid Survival Bible" is an indispensable resource for anyone who wants to embark on a journey of self-sufficiency and resilience, providing all the information needed to live a safe, sustainable and rewarding life off the conventional grid.

# CHAPTER 1.

# INTRODUCTION TO THE BASICS OF OFF-GRID LIVING

## Definition of off-grid living

Off-grid living refers to a lifestyle that is completely self-sufficient and not dependent on utilities such as electricity, water or gas. Those who choose to live off-grid typically generate their own energy through renewable sources such as solar panels or wind turbines, collect rainwater for domestic use, and use alternative methods of waste disposal. This way of living allows individuals to reduce their environmental impact and live more sustainably, minimizing their dependence on fossil fuels and reducing their carbon footprint.

Living off the grid requires a significant amount of planning and preparation. Individuals must carefully consider their energy needs, water consumption and waste management in order to sustain themselves effectively without utilities. This may involve investing in solar panels, water filtration systems and composting toilets, as well as learning essential skills such as gardening, food preservation and conservation. In addition, living off-grid often requires individuals to adopt a simpler, more frugal lifestyle in order to reduce their consumption and make better use of limited resources.

One of the main benefits of off-grid living is the sense of independence and self-sufficiency it provides. By generating their own energy and water, individuals are able to free themselves from the constraints of utilities and reduce their dependence on outside sources for their basic needs. This can be an act of power and liberation, as individuals are no longer beholden to utility companies and are able to control their own resources and infrastructure.

Off-grid living also offers a unique opportunity for individuals to connect with nature and live in harmony with the environment. By relying on renewable energy sources and sustainable practices, off-grid individuals are able to minimize their impact on the planet and their carbon footprint. This way of living can foster a deeper appreciation for the natural world and encourage individuals to live more consciously and consciously in order to preserve the earth for future generations.

However, living off the grid is not without its challenges. Individuals must be prepared for a number of obstacles, including bad weather, limited access to resources, and potential isolation from society. Living off the grid often requires sacrifices and compromises to maintain self-sufficiency, which can be difficult and challenging at times. In addition, living off the grid may not be feasible or practical for everyone, as it requires a certain level of commitment, dedication, and resourcefulness.

Despite the challenges, living off the grid can be a rewarding and enriching experience for those who choose to embrace it. By living off the grid, individuals are able to reduce their environmental impact, live more sustainably, and develop skills essential for self-sufficiency. This way of living offers a unique opportunity to disconnect from the hustle and bustle of modern society and reconnect with nature, while fostering a greater sense of independence and empowerment. Off-grid living may not be for everyone, but for those who are willing to take the challenge, it can be a truly transformative and fulfilling experience.

**Benefits and challenges**

In recent years, its popularity has increased as more people seek to reduce their carbon footprint and gain independence from the grid. While there are numerous benefits to living off-grid, including reduced carbon footprint and lower monthly expenses, there are also significant challenges that need to be addressed. In addition, transitioning to an off-grid lifestyle requires a certain mindset and attitude to be successful.

One of the main benefits of off-grid living is the ability to reduce one's carbon footprint and live a more sustainable lifestyle. By generating their own energy through solar panels or wind turbines, off-grid individuals can significantly reduce their dependence on fossil fuels and lessen their impact on the environment. In addition, off-grid living typically involves the more efficient use of natural resources, such as collecting rainwater for irrigation or installing composting toilets to reduce water waste.

Another key benefit of off-grid living is the potential for lower monthly expenses. By generating their own energy and water, off-grid individuals can eliminate or greatly reduce their utility bills, saving money in the long run. In addition, living off-grid often involves growing one's own food and adopting other sustainable habits, which can lead to further savings on groceries and other expenses.

However, transitioning to an off-grid lifestyle presents a number of challenges. One of the biggest challenges is the upfront cost of setting up off-grid systems, such as purchasing solar panels or installing a septic system. While these costs can be significant up front, they can often be recovered over time through savings on utility bills and other expenses.

Another challenge of off-grid living is the need for a certain level of self-sufficiency and resourcefulness. People who are off-grid must be willing to take on tasks such as repairing their plumbing or troubleshooting problems with their energy systems, as they may not have easy access to professional services. In addition, living off-grid often requires a greater degree of planning and organization, as off-grid individuals must ensure that they have enough food, water and other resources to sustain themselves without depending on outside sources.

In order to successfully make the transition to an off-grid lifestyle, individuals must adopt a certain mindset and attitude. This includes a willingness to embrace a simpler way of living and prioritize self-sufficiency over convenience. Living off-grid often requires a willingness to make sacrifices and adapt to new ways of doing things, such as using renewable energy sources or collecting rainwater for household use.

In addition, off-grid individuals must commit to continually learning and improving their self-sufficiency skills. This may involve courses on sustainable living practices, attending workshops on renewable energy systems, or connecting with other off-grid individuals to share knowledge and resources. By staying informed and actively seeking new information, off-grid individuals can ensure that they are prepared for any challenges that may arise.

While off-grid living offers many benefits, it also presents unique challenges that must be overcome. Successfully transitioning to an off-grid lifestyle requires a certain mindset, including a willingness to embrace sustainability, self-sufficiency, and continuous learning. By meeting these challenges with determination and perseverance, off-grid individuals can reap the benefits of a more sustainable and independent way of life.

HAPTER 2.

WATER RESOURCES

Water is an essential natural resource vital to all living organisms on Earth. It plays a crucial role in maintaining the balance of ecosystems and sustaining life. The availability of clean and safe water is an urgent issue in many parts of the world, as access to clean water is important for human health and well-being. Therefore, water resource management, harvesting, well construction, and natural water sources are important aspects of water sustainability and conservation.

Water resources refer to all sources of water available for use, including rivers, lakes, groundwater and precipitation. Water resources management involves ensuring the sustainability of water supplies for future generations. This includes monitoring water quality, regulating its use, and implementing strategies to protect water sources from contamination. In addition, efforts should be made to promote water conservation and reduce waste to ensure efficient use of water resources.

Water harvesting involves the process of collecting and storing water for various uses. This may include rainwater harvesting, surface water harvesting from rivers and lakes, or groundwater extraction from wells. Appropriate collection methods are essential to ensure the availability of clean and safe water for drinking, irrigation and other purposes. In addition, effective water harvesting systems can help mitigate the impact of drought and water scarcity in water-scarce regions.

Well construction is an important aspect of water management, especially in areas where groundwater is the primary source of water. Wells are typically drilled or dug into the ground to access groundwater sources, such as aquifers. The construction of a well is essential to ensure the quality and quantity of groundwater extracted. This includes selecting suitable locations, using appropriate drilling techniques, and installing well casings to prevent contamination of the water supply.

Natural water sources, such as rivers, lakes and wetlands, play a crucial role in providing water for human consumption and sustaining biodiversity. These ecosystems are home to a wide variety of plant and animal species, and play a vital role in regulating the water cycle and maintaining water quality. Protecting natural water sources from pollution and overuse is essential to ensure their continued availability and ecological health. Efforts must be made to conserve these valuable resources for future generations.

Effective management of water resources is essential to ensure the availability of clean and safe water for all living organisms on Earth. Through the implementation of appropriate water management practices, such as promoting water conservation, monitoring water quality and protecting natural water sources, we can work toward a more sustainable future of water resources. It is important that individuals, communities and governments work together and take action to safeguard water sources and ensure their longevity for generations to come.

With the increase in pollution and contamination of water sources, it has become crucial to have effective methods for water purification and filtration. In this essay, we will discuss three common methods of water purification and filtration - solar stills, chemical treatment, and filtration.

Solar stills are a simple and effective way to purify water using the energy of the sun. Solar stills work by using the heat of the sun to evaporate water, leaving behind impurities and contaminants. The purified water condenses on a surface and can be collected for drinking. Solar stills are particularly useful in remote areas with limited access to clean water sources, as they do not require electricity or fuel to operate.

Chemical treatment is another common method of water purification and filtration. Chemicals such as chlorine, iodine and ozone are commonly used to disinfect water and kill harmful bacteria and pathogens. These chemicals work by breaking down the cell walls of micro-organisms, making them harmless. Chemical treatment is effective in killing a wide range of contaminants, but it can leave a chemical taste and smell in the water, which some people may find unpleasant.

Filtration is a mechanical method of water purification and filtration that works by passing the water through a physical barrier to remove impurities. Different types of filters are available, including activated carbon filters, ceramic filters and reverse osmosis filters. Activated carbon filters work by adsorbing organic compounds and chemicals, while ceramic filters work by trapping bacteria and pathogens in the tiny pores of the filter material. Reverse osmosis filters use a semi-permeable membrane to remove contaminants from the water by forcing it through the membrane under pressure.

Each of these methods has its own advantages and disadvantages. Solar stills are cheap and easy to use, but they can be slow and inefficient in purifying large amounts of water. Chemical treatment is effective in killing a wide range of contaminants, but it can leave a chemical taste and smell in the water. Filtration is an effective mechanical method for removing a wide range of impurities, but it can be expensive and require regular maintenance.

Each method has its strengths and weaknesses, and the best

method will depend on factors such as cost, resource availability and level of contamination in the water source. By understanding the different methods of water purification and filtration, we can ensure that everyone has access to clean and safe drinking water.

**Water Sources**

Water availability is critical for off-grid survival. The main water sources include rainwater, wells and natural watercourses such as rivers and lakes. Each source has its advantages and disadvantages, and the choice will depend on location and available resources. The identification and development of a reliable source of water supply is the first crucial step in ensuring a continuous and secure supply of this essential element.

- Main sources of water supply
- Rivers: Streams flowing into oceans, lakes or other rivers
- Ponds and ponds: small bodies of stagnant or near-stagnant water
- Lakes: Large bodies of stagnant water, often of natural or man-made origin
- Sources: Points where groundwater naturally emerges to the

surface
- Wells: Digging or drilling in the ground to extract groundwater
- Ruscelletti and torrents: Small streams that flow generally in mountainous or hilly areas
- Glaciers: Permanent ice masses that release water through melting
- Aquifers: Permeable rock layers containing water

**Natural fountains**

- Water jets from the ground, often intermittently: Groundwater
- Water flows below the earth's surface
- Rainwater: Water collected from rain, often used through collection systems
- Lagoons: Brackish water basins separated from the sea by sandbars or coral reefs

**Swamps**

- Areas of soil saturated with water, often with aquatic vegetation
- Estuaries: Transition zones where fresh water from rivers meets salt water from the sea
- Aquifers: Rock strata or water-saturated permeable sediments, which may be accessible through wells or springs
- Melting water: Water derived from melting snow or ice, especially in spring and summer

## Collection of Rainwater

Rainwater harvesting is an efficient and sustainable technique to ensure a source of water. Using gutter and reservoir systems, rainwater can be collected and stored for domestic and agricultural use. This method requires an initial investment in equipment such as gutters, filters and tanks but can significantly reduce dependence on other sources. It is important to ensure that the water collected is treated properly to avoid contamination.

## Construction of wells

Wells are a vital source of water for those living off-grid. The construction of a well requires a geological assessment to detect the presence of aquifers. There are different types of wells, including hand-dug and drilled wells. The choice depends on the depth of water and the resources available. The wells are protected from contamination by appropriate covers and regularly maintained to ensure continuous and safe supply.

## Use of natural watercourses

Natural watercourses, such as rivers and lakes, can provide an abundant source of water but require special attention to ensure their safety. It is essential to analyse the quality of water and install filtration systems to remove impurities and pathogens.

Also, the use of pumps may be necessary to transport water from the watercourse to your home. Sustainable management of natural water resources is essential to avoid over-exploitation and contamination.

## Water Treatment

Water purification is crucial to ensuring that it is safe to drink. Even clean water sources may contain invisible contaminants. There are various methods to purify water, each with its own advantages and limitations.

## Filtrfation Methods

Filtration is one of the most common methods for purifying water. Activated carbon filters can remove organic impurities, chlorine and some heavy metals. Membrane filters, such as reverse osmosis filters, are effective in removing bacteria, viruses and other fine particles. The installation of a suitable filtration system requires an assessment of the specific needs and quality of the available water.

## Solar Alembics

Solar stills use the energy of the sun to purify water through evaporation and condensation. This method is particularly useful in sunny areas and can be built using simple materials such as glass, plastic and metal. Water is heated by the sun, evaporating and leaving behind solid contaminants, then condensing into a purified form. This process is slow, but very effective in removing a wide range of impurities.

**Chemical treatment**

Chemical treatment, using substances such as chlorine or iodine, is a quick and effective method of purifying water, especially in emergency situations. These chemicals can kill bacteria, viruses and other harmful micro-organisms. However, it is important to follow the dosage instructions carefully to avoid excessive exposure to chemicals. Chemical treatment is often used in combination with other purification methods to ensure maximum water safety.

**Water storage and conservation**

Once obtained and purified, the water must be stored in an appropriate manner to avoid future contamination. Storage tanks shall be cleaned regularly and protected from external contamination. It is important to use suitable materials such as food-grade plastic or stainless steel to prevent harmful substances from seeping into the water. Also, keeping water in closed containers and away from direct sunlight can prevent the growth of algae and bacteria.

Effective water management is essential for a sustainable and safe life outside the grid. From collection to purification, each phase must be carefully planned and monitored to ensure a continuous supply of clean and safe water.

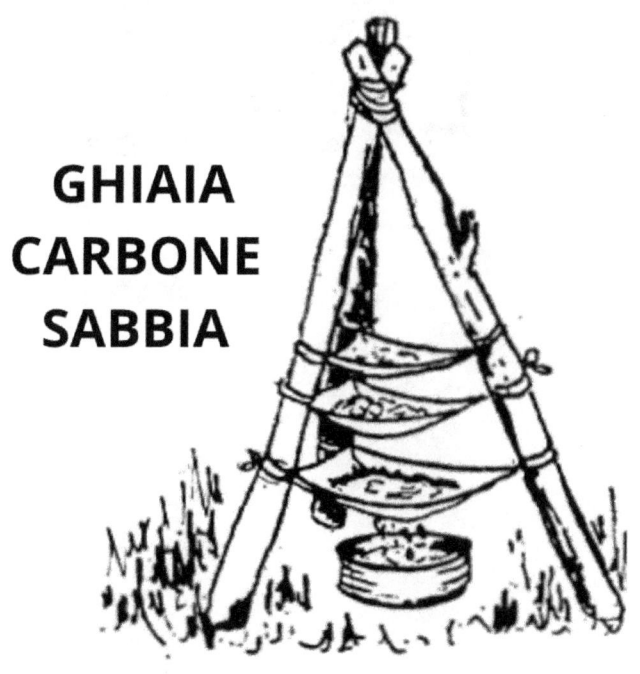

**GHIAIA**
**CARBONE**
**SABBIA**

**GHIAIA**
**SABBIA**
**CARBONE**
**GHIAIA**

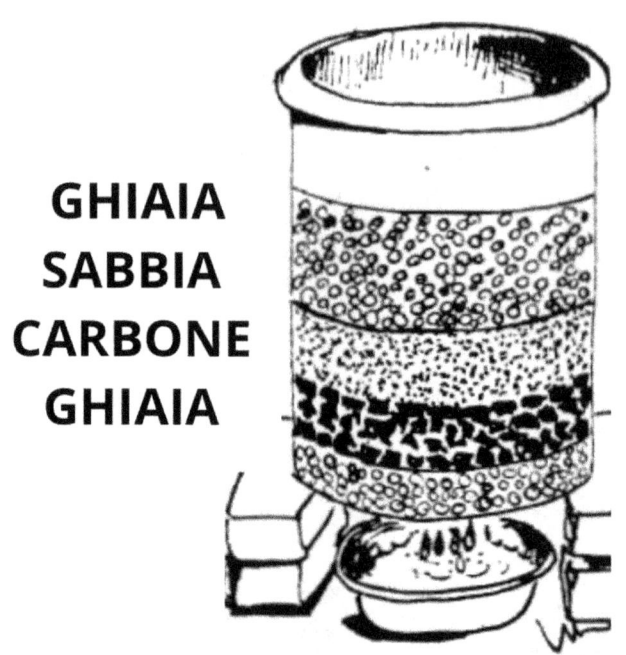

# Sistema completo di raccolta e distribuzione

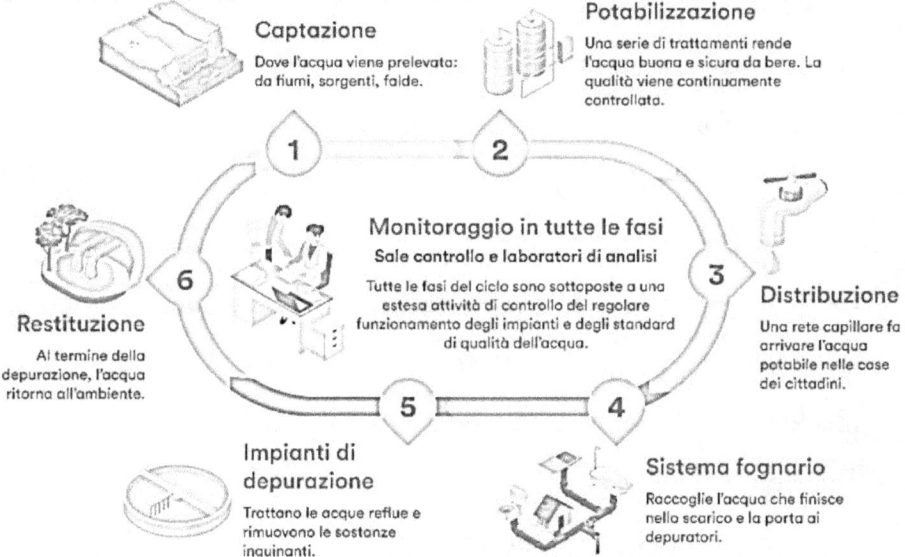

# CHAPTER 3.

## FOOD SUSTAINABILITY

### Food production

One of the main competitive trends in maternal and primary education is the increasing emphasis on technological integration. Schools are incorporating technology into their classrooms to improve learning experiences and prepare students for the digital age. This includes providing students with access to devices such as tablets and laptops, as well as using online learning platforms and educational apps. Schools that can effectively integrate technology into their curriculum are often seen as more attractive options by parents seeking a modern and innovative educational experience for their children.

Another competitive trend in maternal and primary education is an increasing focus on individualized and personalized learning. Parents are increasingly looking for schools that meet the unique needs and abilities of each child, rather than a single educational approach for all. Schools that are able to offer personalised learning plans, Small classes and differentiated education are often seen as more attractive options for parents seeking educational opportunities in line with their children's specific learning styles and interests.

In addition to technological advances and personalized learning, another competitive trend in maternal and primary education is the emphasis on holistic development. Schools must be able to provide a comprehensive education that goes beyond the academic aspects to include social, emotional and physical development. Schools offering a wide range of extracurricular activities, such as sports, music, arts and community services, are often seen as more attractive options for parents seeking a full education for their children.

The increasing globalization of education is another competitive trend affecting nursery and primary schools. Schools are recognising the importance of exposing students to different perspectives and cultures in order to prepare them for a globalised world. As a result, schools are incorporating international study programmes, language programmes and cultural exchange opportunities into their offerings. Schools that can offer students international experiences and perspectives are often seen as more competitive options by parents seeking a truly global education for their children.

The rise of alternative educational models, such as Montessori, Waldorf and Reggio Emilia, is another competitive trend in maternal and primary education. Parents are increasingly choosing schools that offer alternative approaches to education that focus on creativity, self-directed learning and hands-on experiences. Schools that can offer students unique and innovative educational philosophies are often seen as more attractive options for parents seeking an untraditional educational experience for their children.

The growing competition between nursery and primary schools to attract and retain students is driving a trend towards more marketing and branding efforts. Schools are investing in professional marketing strategies, such as social media campaigns, website development and targeted advertising, to differentiate themselves in a crowded market. Schools that are able to effectively communicate their unique value propositions and show their strengths often succeed better in attracting new students and retaining existing ones.

A competitive and rapidly evolving educational landscape that requires them to adapt to changing trends to remain relevant and meet the needs of students and parents. Embracing technological integration, personalized learning, holistic development, globalization, alternative educational models and enhanced marketing efforts, schools can position themselves as competitive options in the education market. It is crucial that schools stay informed about current trends and continuously innovate in order to provide high quality educational experiences that set them apart from the competition.

Food production is a key pillar for sustainable and self-sufficient life outside the grid. This process involves the cultivation of vegetables, fruits, cereals and livestock. The key to effective food production is the diversification of crops and techniques, to ensure balanced nutrition and resilience against adverse weather conditions and pests.

One of the most effective techniques in food production is crop rotation. This method avoids soil depletion and reduces the incidence of specific plant diseases and pests. In addition, the use of compost and organic fertilizers improves soil fertility by promoting healthy plant growth. Animal husbandry, such as chickens, goats, and rabbits, provides essential protein and other products such as eggs, milk, and wool. Animals can also contribute to soil fertilization through manure.

Crop selection is crucial. Growing disease-resistant local varieties increases the chances of success. Perennial plants, which grow back every year without the need for replanting, are particularly useful in a self-sustaining system. In addition, the integration of medicinal and aromatic plants can improve overall health and well-being.

Food production also requires effective management of water resources. Efficient irrigation systems, such as drip irrigation, can reduce water consumption and ensure that plants receive the necessary moisture. Collection and storage of rainwater in reservoirs is a common practice to ensure a constant supply of water, especially during drought periods.

## Permaculture and sustainable agriculture

Permaculture and sustainable agriculture are integrated approaches to food production that aim at creating stable and sustainable agricultural ecosystems. Permaculture, in particular, is based on ecological design principles that mimic patterns and relationships found in natural ecosystems.

One of the fundamental principles of permaculture is the efficient use of resources. This includes wastewater collection and re-use, composting of bio-waste and implementation of natural construction techniques. Permaculture promotes biodiversity and the use of perennial plants, which require less maintenance than annual crops.

Sustainable agriculture, on the other hand, focuses on the use of agricultural practices that protect the environment, support public health, and promote social and economic justice. Techniques such as cross-cropping, where different plants are grown together to improve soil health and reduce pest pressure, are examples of sustainable practices.

Another crucial aspect of permaculture is observation and interaction with the environment. This approach allows crop techniques to be adapted to specific climatic and geographical conditions, improving efficiency and productivity. Permaculture also encourages the creation of community support networks, where knowledge and resources are shared to promote collective sustainability.

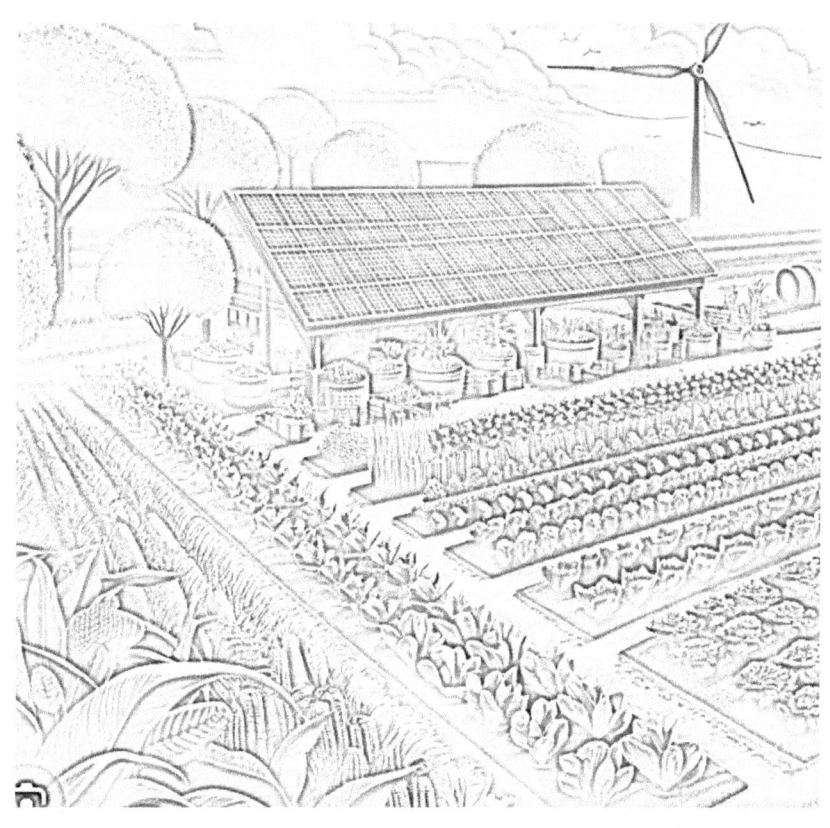

## Gardening in small spaces

Small-space gardening is a practical and versatile solution for food production, particularly useful for those living in urban areas or with limited access to arable land. This practice can be carried out on balconies, terraces and even inside houses, using techniques such as vertical gardening, containers and raised beds.

Vertical gardening uses vertical surfaces to grow plants, maximizing the use of space. This can be achieved by using grids, recycled pallets, PVC pipes or prefabricated modular systems. Vines such as tomatoes and cucumbers are particularly suitable for these systems. Herbs and leafy vegetables can also thrive in vertical gardens, offering a bountiful harvest in a small space.

The use of containers is another effective technique. Pots, crates and other types of containers can be used to grow a wide range of plants. The containers can be easily moved to optimize exposure to sunlight and protect them from adverse weather conditions. It is important to choose containers with good drainage and use high quality soil to ensure the health of the plants.

Raised beds are structures that raise the growing ground above the surrounding soil level, improving drainage and facilitating land management. These beds can be constructed using materials such as wood, brick or concrete blocks. They provide a controlled growing environment, which can be enriched with compost and other soil improvers to improve soil fertility.

**Growing fruit trees**

Growing fruit trees is a sustainable and productive practice that can provide a continuous source of fresh, nutritious fruit. Fruit trees require careful planning and constant management, but the long-term benefits include abundant harvests and increased self-sufficiency.

Before planting, it is crucial to select the varieties of fruit trees that are suitable for the local climate and soil. Some trees, such as citrus trees, require warm and sunny climates, while others, such as apple orchards, can thrive in colder climates. The choice of disease and pest-resistant varieties can reduce the need for chemical intervention.

Soil preparation is crucial for the health of fruit trees. The soil must be well-drained and rich in organic matter. Adding compost and other soil improvers can improve soil structure and provide essential nutrients. Planting trees should be done following species-specific guidelines, making sure the roots have enough room to expand.

Once planted, fruit trees require regular care. Irrigation is essential, especially during drought periods. Annual pruning helps to maintain the shape of the tree, improve air circulation, and stimulate fruit production. The fight against diseases and pests is also important, using biological and integrated methods to minimize environmental impact.

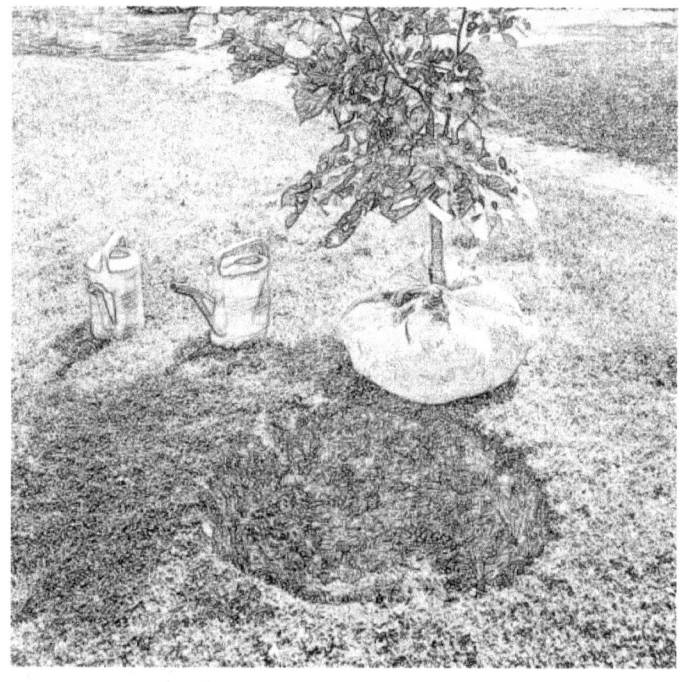

## Food supply

Food supply includes traditional methods such as hunting, fishing and gathering of wild plants. These practices can complement food production by providing proteins and nutrients that might be difficult to obtain with agriculture alone. Hunting requires specific skills and a thorough knowledge of the local ecosystem. It is essential to comply with local laws and regulations, as well as practicing ethical and sustainable hunting techniques. Traps can be used to capture small animals, but they must be placed and monitored carefully to avoid unnecessary suffering to the animals.

Fishing is another valuable source of food. It can be practiced in rivers, lakes and seas using a variety of equipment and techniques. Sustainable fishing means selecting unexploited species and respecting catch quotas to ensure the conservation of fish stocks.

The collection of edible wild plants requires a thorough knowledge of the local flora. Some plants can be harvested in the wild and used as a food source, but it is essential to know how to distinguish between edible and toxic species. Harvesting must be carried out sustainably, avoiding damage to the ecosystem and ensuring the regeneration of plants.

### Storage of food

Food preservation is essential to ensure a continuous supply of food, especially in times of scarcity. There are various methods of preservation, including canning, dehydration, smoking, fermentation and vinegar.

### Storage in cans

Canning is an effective method of preserving fruit, vegetables, and meat. This process involves heating food at high temperatures to destroy harmful micro-organisms, followed by sealing the food in airtight containers. It is important to follow safety guidelines to prevent the risk of botulism and other contamination.

### Dehydration and smoking

Dehydration removes moisture from food, preventing the growth of mold and bacteria. This method is ideal for fruits, vegetables, herbs and meat. Smoking uses smoke to preserve and flavor meat and fish. Both methods require specific equipment, such as tumblers and smokers, as well as knowledge of appropriate techniques.

### Fermentation and Vinegar

Fermentation is a preservation method that uses beneficial bacteria to process and preserve food. This process can improve the nutritional value and digestibility of food. Common examples include sauerkraut, kimchi and yogurt. Vinegar, on the other hand, uses acetic acid in vinegar to preserve vegetables and fruits, creating unique flavors and extending shelf life.

Food sustainability in the off-grid context requires an integrated and diversified approach to food production and conservation. By implementing these practices, it is possible to ensure a continuous and secure food supply, reducing dependence on external resources and promoting a self-sufficient lifestyle.

## Permaculture and Sustainable Agriculture

Design of agricultural systems:
- Creating agricultural ecosystems that mimic nature

Integrated land management:
Use of compost and mulch to improve soil health

Water conservation:
- Rainwater harvesting techniques and efficient irrigation

Biodiversity:
- Growing a variety of plants to prevent diseases and pests

Crop rotation: The
- Alternating crops to maintain soil fertility

Integrated livestock farming:
- Integration of animals for bio-waste management and soil fertilization

Sustainable forestry:
- Forest management for timber and food products without degrading the ecosystem

## Gardening in Small Spaces

Vertical gardens:

- Growing plants on vertical structures to save space

Containers and jars:

- Use of containers to grow plants on balconies and terraces

Table of cultivation:

- Raised tables for intensive and ergonomic horticulture

Intercropping techniques:

- Growing more plant species in the same space to optimise land use

Use of mini-greenhouses:

- Small greenhouses to extend the growing season and protect plants

Aquaponics gardens:

- Combined plant and fish farming systems

**Urban gardens:**

**Small green areas used for growing vegetables and flowers**

### Growing fruit trees

Selection of species:
- Choice of trees suitable for the local climate

Correct planting:
- Soil preparation and planting at the right depth

Regular pruning:
- Pruning to maintain healthy and productive trees

Efficient irrigation:
- Irrigation systems to provide water without waste

Pest control:
- Use of natural methods to protect trees from pests

Organic fertiliser: The
- Use of compost and natural fertilizers to feed trees

Pollination: The
- Encourage pollination with the help of bees and other beneficial insects

## Examples of Permaculture and Sustainable Agriculture

Example: A farm using permaculture techniques could have a herb garden near the house, a diversified vegetable garden, and a small orchard, Integrated animals such as chickens and goats for bio-waste management and soil fertilization.

## Gardening in Small Spaces

Example: A city apartment with a balcony transformed into a vertical garden with tomato plants, herbs, and strawberries grown in hanging pots and vertical shelves. A small aquaponics system in the living room could grow lettuce and fish.

## Growing fruit trees

Example: A home garden with apple, pear and cherry trees planted in the correct spacing, regularly pruned, watered with a drip system, and treated with biological remedies against pests to ensure an abundant and healthy production of fruit each year.

## Procuring Food

Hunting and Trapping

Types of hunting:
- Hunting with bow and arrows
- Hunting with firearms
- Hunting with primitive weapons (spears, boomerangs, etc.)
- Hunting with hunting dogs

### Hunting Techniques:
- Hunting in the background
- Hunting and pursuit
- Hunting with recall
- Hunting with the use of hiding places

### Types of Traps:
- Fall traps (stones, logs)
- Snare traps (with wire or rope)
- Spring traps
- Traps with covered holes
- Cage traps

### Legislation and ethics:
- Know the local hunting laws
- Ethical and sustainable hunting practices
- Evisceration techniques and food preparation

## Fisheries and aquaculture

Tipi di Pesca:
- Fishing with rods
- Fishing with nets
- Underwater fishing
- Fishing with fish traps
- Fishing with harriers

## Fishing techniques:
- Freshwater fishing (rivers, lakes, ponds)
- Saltwater fishing (sea, ocean)
- Fishing with live or artificial lures
- Fly fishing

## Aquaculture:
- Fish farming in ponds or reservoirs
- Farming of mollusks (oysters, mussels)
- Shellfish farming (shrimps, crabs)
- Management and maintenance of aquaculture facilities
- Feeding and care techniques for aquatic animals

## Legislation and ethics:
- Know the local fishing laws
- Sustainable fishing practices and quota compliance
- Collection of Edible Wild Plants

## Types of Edible Plants:
- Herbs (nettle, dandelion, yarrow)
- Berries (blueberries, raspberries, blackberries)
- Mushrooms (porcini, chanterelles, nails)
- Roots and tubers (horseradish, burdock)
- Edible flowers (violets, pumpkin flowers)
- Leaves and sprouts (wild spinach, fern sprouts)

## Collection Techniques:
Correct identification of plants

Seasonal harvesting and rotation of collection areas

Sustainable harvesting techniques to avoid depletion of resources

Collected in uncontaminated places (away from busy roads, industries, etc.)

## Preparation and storage:
- Cleaning and preparation of harvested plants
- Preservation techniques (drying, freezing, canning)

## Legislation and ethics:
- Know the local laws on wild plant harvesting
- Ethical harvesting practices to preserve the ecosystem
- Education on ecological awareness and respect for nature

# How to store food

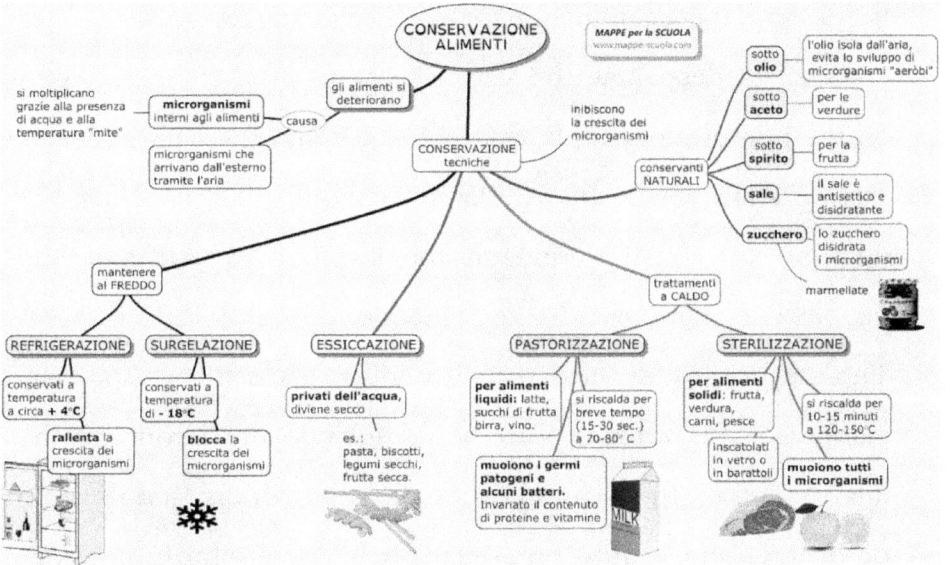

# CHAPTER 4.

## CONSTRUCTION OF SHELTERS

### Planning the shelter

Shelter planning is the first crucial step to building a functional and safe facility. This phase includes the definition of housing needs and the examination of local climatic conditions. It is essential to determine the size and layout of the shelter based on the number of people who will use it and the daily activities that will take place there. Planning should also consider the duration of construction and the level of expertise of the people involved.

The creation of detailed sketches and plans is a key aspect of planning. This information should include the layout of the interior spaces, the location of windows and doors, and the type of heating and ventilation system. It is also useful to consider the resources needed and construction techniques best suited to the context. Using design software can make it easier to view and edit plans, ensuring that every detail is considered before you start construction.

## Choice of location

The choice of location is crucial for the safety and effectiveness of the shelter. Ideally, the site should be located in a high and well-drained area to avoid flooding and water infiltration. Proximity to natural resources such as wood, water and building materials is beneficial, but it is equally important to assess exposure to the elements. A shelter should be built in a location that minimizes the impact of strong winds, heavy rain, and heavy snow.

It is also important to consider the prevailing wind direction and exposure to the sun. A well-oriented location can maximize energy efficiency by improving the shelter's ability to maintain a comfortable temperature. In addition, the chosen site must comply with all local building rules and regulations to ensure that construction is legal and safe.

## Evaluation of local resources

The assessment of local resources is essential for the construction of the shelter. This phase involves the analysis of available materials in the vicinity and their suitability for the project. Wood, stone, and mud are common resources, but their quality and availability may vary. It is useful to map local resources, including the sustainability and environmental impact of materials extraction.

The assessment of resources includes the availability of water for the treatment of materials and works. It is also important to consider the accessibility of resources and how easily they can be transported to the site. Sustainable management of local resources can reduce costs and minimize the environmental impact of the project.

**Building materials**

The choice of building materials directly affects the durability, energy efficiency and comfort of the shelter. Traditional materials such as wood and stone offer strength and insulation, but they must be treated and maintained properly to ensure their longevity. Wood is ideal for the supporting structure and decorative elements, while stone can be used for foundations and walls.

Other materials include mud and earth, which offer excellent thermal insulation properties and can be used in such constructions as terracotta houses or mud houses. It is important to select materials that are suitable for local climatic conditions and offer a good cost-benefit ratio.

**Land use and mud**

Earth and mud are traditional materials that can be used to build strong, well-insulated shelters. Clay and mud bricks are known for their thermal and acoustic insulation properties. These materials can be processed locally, reducing costs and environmental impact.

Construction with soil and mud requires specific techniques such as the construction of sack walls and the use of clay and sand to improve cohesion and stability. It is essential to make sure the materials are well dry before use to avoid problems of moisture and deterioration over time. In addition, the application of protective finishes can extend the service life and improve weathering resistance

**Wood and stone**

Wood and stone are traditional materials widely used in the construction of shelters, thanks to their durability and versatility. When treated properly, wood can serve as a supporting structure, external and internal cladding, as well as decorative elements. It offers excellent insulation properties and good resistance to the elements but requires regular maintenance to avoid insect damage and moisture.

Stone, on the other hand, is particularly suitable for foundations, walls and fireplaces. It offers intrinsic strength and exceptional resistance to fire and moisture. Stone constructions, such as dry-type ones, do not require mortar and can be very durable over time. Both materials require specific skills in processing and laying to ensure a stable and safe construction.

## Recycled and renewable materials

The use of recycled and renewable materials in shelter construction is an environmentally friendly approach that contributes to sustainability and waste reduction. Recycled materials such as metal, glass and demolition wood can be re-used to build robust and functional structures. This approach not only reduces the demand for new resources but also decreases the environmental impact of construction.

Renewable materials such as bamboo and cork offer sustainable solutions for buildings. Bamboo is particularly known for its rapid growth and strength, while cork, derived from the bark of cork oak, is an excellent natural insulator. The use of renewable materials helps to maintain ecological balance and promotes sustainable construction practices.

## Design and construction

The design and construction of a shelter require careful planning and an in-depth knowledge of construction techniques. The design shall take into account the use of materials, the layout of spaces, and specific housing requirements. Construction techniques must be adapted to the available resources and environmental conditions.

It is important to follow the best construction practices to ensure the quality and durability of the shelter. This includes the proper preparation of the site, the use of appropriate tools and techniques, and compliance with safety principles. Construction must be done accurately, following design plans and making sure each step of the process is completed correctly to avoid future problems.

**Traditional construction techniques**
Traditional construction techniques offer proven solutions for the construction of durable and functional shelters. These techniques, often passed down from generation to generation, include methods such as dry construction, the use of mud and earth walls, and wood weaving.
Dry construction uses stones laid without mortar to create strong and stable walls. This method is particularly useful in areas with an abundance of stones and can be achieved using simple techniques and local materials. The use of mud and earth walls, as in cob or rammed earth methods, offers excellent insulation properties and can be adapted to various architectural styles.

**Insulation and energy efficiency**
Insulation and energy efficiency are key to ensuring the comfort and sustainability of a shelter. Good insulation reduces heat loss

during the winter and maintains freshness during the summer. The use of natural insulation materials, such as wood fiber, wool or hemp, can significantly improve the energy efficiency of the shelter.

The design should also consider the orientation of the shelter to maximize passive solar gain. The insertion of strategic windows and openings can improve natural ventilation and reduce the need for mechanical heating and cooling. The use of techniques such as closed air design and heat recovery can further optimise energy efficiency.

**Integration of ventilation systems**

The integration of ventilation systems is essential to ensure health and comfort within a shelter. Proper ventilation prevents moisture build-up, reduces the risk of mold, and improves indoor air quality. Ventilation systems may be natural, mechanical or a combination of both depending on the specific needs of the shelter and available resources.

Natural ventilation uses the principles of passive architecture, such as strategic arrangement of windows, doors and openings. Cross ventilation, which consists of placing windows or openings on opposite sides of the shelter, promotes air flow and natural cooling. Air inlets and vents, located at high points, allow the hot air to escape while the lower openings facilitate the entry of fresh air.

To improve the efficiency of natural ventilation, devices such as natural flow fans or solar fans can be installed, They use solar energy to improve air circulation without the use of external electricity. These fans can be integrated into ceilings or walls to optimize air flow in all seasons.

## Planning the Shelter
## Choice of Location
### Ground

- Prefer stable and well-drained soil
- Avoid areas prone to flooding, landslides or avalanches
- Consider sun exposure for natural heating

### Proximity to natural resources

- Proximity to water sources (rivers, lakes, springs)
- Presence of natural building materials (wood, stone, earth)

### Accessibility

- Easy access for material transport and maintenance
- Distance from main roads and trails for safety and privacy

### Protection against the elements
- Natural shelter from wind, snow and rain (hills, trees)
- Orientation of the shelter to maximize protection

### Wildlife
- Consider the presence of wild animals for safety
- Location away from dens or animal paths to avoid conflicts

### Evaluation of local resources
### Building materials
### Wood:
- Availability of suitable trees (conifers, broadleaved)
- Assessment of the health of trees (absence of disease or rot)

### Stone:
- Presence of easily workable rocks (limestone, sandstone)
- Accessibility of stones without damaging the environment

### Earth:
- Soil quality for clay or mud brick construction
- Availability of clay for plastering and bricks

### Water
- Drinking water sources nearby
- Accessibility for the construction of rainwater collection systems

### Plants and vegetation
- Use of local plants for roof vegetation

- Useful plants for the production of fibers and ropes (hemp, nettle)

**Local Climate**

- Seasonal average temperatures to determine insulation requirements

**Annual rainfall to design drainage system**

**Renewable Energy**

- Potential for solar energy (exposure to the sun)
- Wind potential (prevailing winds)
- Water sources for small hydroelectric plants

## Example 1: Wooden shelter

Planning and preparation

Location: In a clearing near a stream, with plenty of pine trees.

Local Resource Assessment: Availability of timber, foundation stones, and clay for plaster.

Materials Needed

Pine logs

Stones for the foundation

Clay and sand for plaster

Nails and screws

Wooden roof tiles for the roof

Recycled glass windows

Construction

Foundations: Dig a trench for the foundation and fill it with stones. Cover with a mixture of clay and sand to stabilize.

Structure: Cut pine logs and build the walls with the technique of dovetail interlocking. Fix with nails.

Roof: Make a truss structure and cover it with wooden tiles. Make sure the roof is tilted to let water drain.

Floor: Cover the ground with a base of stones and add a floor of wooden boards.

Windows and Door: Install recycled glass windows and a wooden door.

## Example 2: Shelter in Earth and Straw

### Planning and preparation

Location: On a slight slope to facilitate water drainage.

Local Resource Assessment: Abundance of clay, sand and straw.

Materials Needed

Clay

Sand

Straw

Wooden branches for the structure

Stones for the foundation

Glass bottles for windows

Tarpaulin for the roof

Construction

Foundations: Dig a trench and fill it with stones for a stable base.

Structure: Create a basic structure with strong branches.

Walls: Mix clay, sand, and straw to create adobe bricks. Build the walls with these bricks.

Roof: Build a wooden structure and cover with tarpaulin, covered by a layer of earth for insulation.

Windows and Door: Use glass bottles embedded in the walls for the windows and build a wooden door.

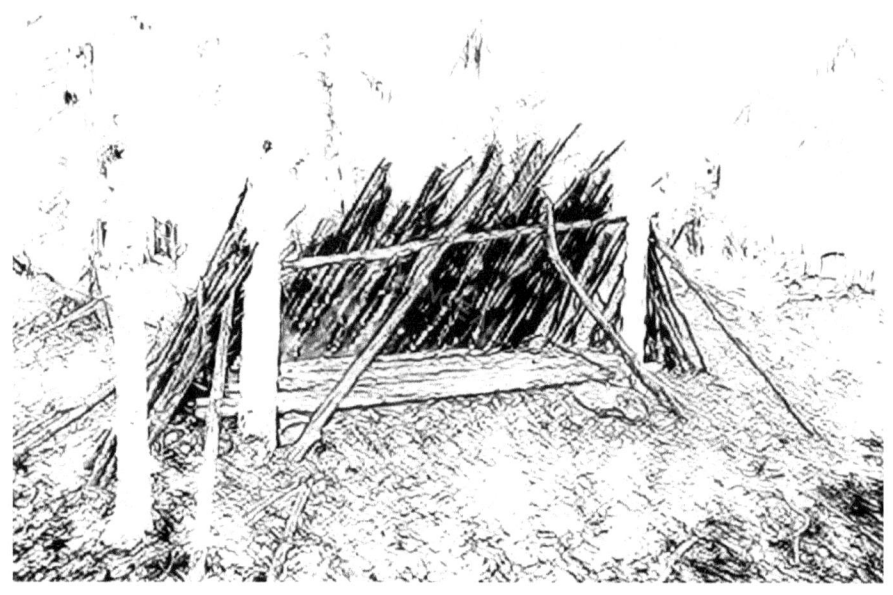

CAPITOLO 5.

ENERGIA RINNOVABILE

**Overview of Renewable Energy Options**

Renewable energy is a sustainable and environmentally friendly solution to meeting energy needs, reducing dependence on fossil fuels and reducing greenhouse gas emissions. The main renewable energy options include solar, wind and hydro, each with its own specific characteristics and advantages.

Solar energy uses solar radiation to generate electricity through photovoltaic panels or to produce heat through thermal solar collectors. It is one of the most popular renewable energy sources due to its global availability and ability to be implemented in small and large scale.

Wind energy uses the wind to run turbines and generate electricity. This technology is particularly effective in areas with constant winds and can be installed both on land and at sea. Wind turbines offer a clean, low-cost energy option once installed.

Hydropower uses the movement of water, such as rivers or waterfalls, to produce energy. Hydroelectric systems range from large dams to smaller installations called micro-hydro-electric. This energy source is particularly useful in regions with abundant water resources.

**Solar**

Solar energy is one of the most affordable and growing renewable energy sources. Solar photovoltaic panels convert sunlight into electricity through silicon cells that generate direct current when exposed to sunlight. These panels can be installed on roofs, land or special structures and are suitable for both residential and commercial applications.

There are two main types of solar systems: photovoltaic and thermal. Photovoltaic systems generate electricity which can be used to power electrical devices and heat water, solar thermal systems are designed to heat water directly through solar collectors.

The effectiveness of a solar system depends on the amount of sunlight it receives, which can vary depending on its geographical location and weather conditions. Maintenance of solar panels is generally simple, requiring only periodic cleaning to remove dust and debris that can reduce efficiency.

The installation of solar panels involves choosing a suitable site that receives sufficient sunlight. Panels should be mounted on an inclined or horizontal surface with the optimal orientation and angle of inclination to maximize exposure to the sun. It is essential to install the panels safely and ensure a proper electrical connection to the storage system or power grid.

Maintenance of solar panels includes regular cleaning of

surfaces to remove dust and debris that may reduce efficiency. It is also important to monitor the system via inverters and other equipment to detect any problems or performance drops. Electrical components must be checked periodically to ensure that there are no leaks or short circuits.

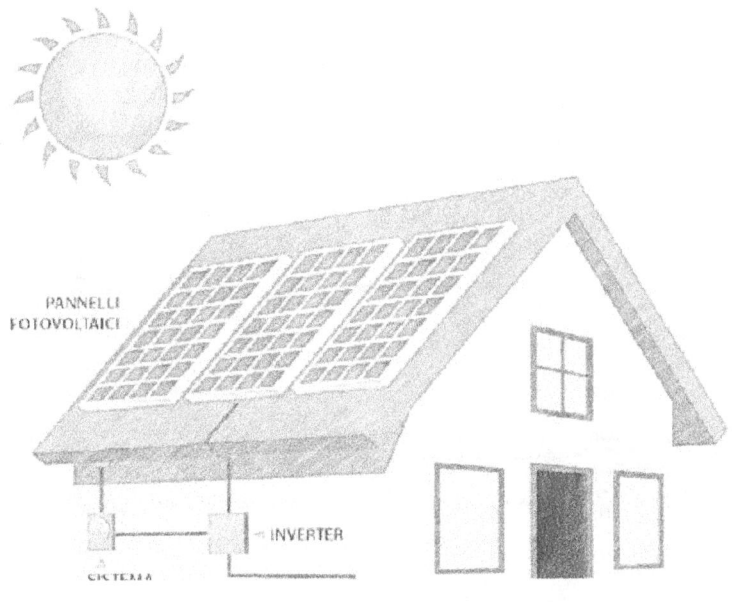

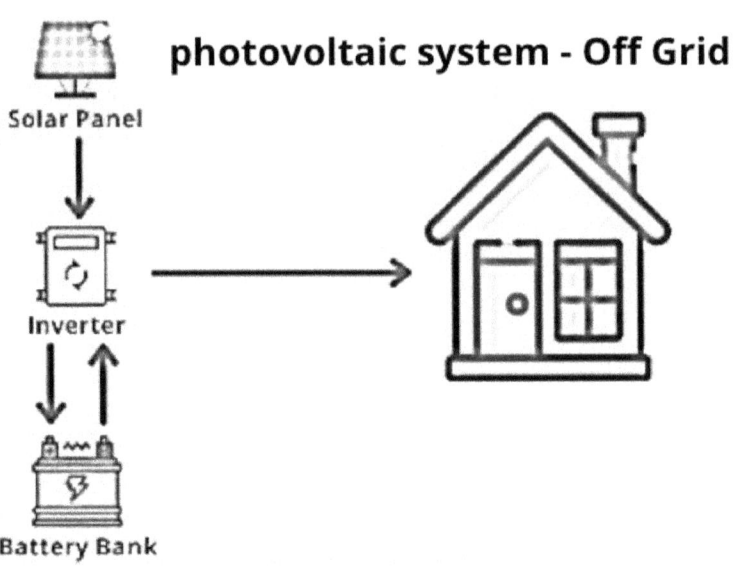

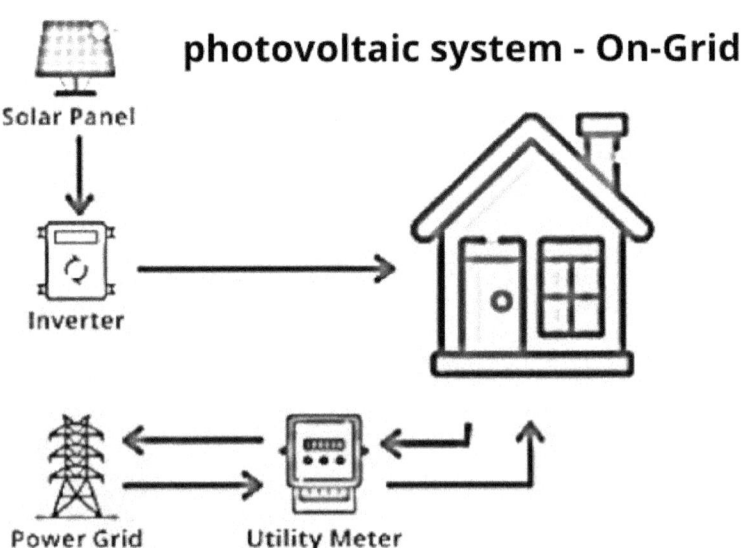

Wind energy uses the force of the wind to generate electricity through wind turbines. These turbines, equipped with rotating blades, convert the kinetic energy of the wind into mechanical energy and then electricity. Wind turbines can be installed onshore (onshore) or offshore (offshore), depending on the available wind resources and specific requirements.

Onshore wind installations are generally cheaper and easier to maintain than their offshore counterparts. However, offshore turbines can capture stronger and more constant winds, resulting in higher energy production. Wind turbines must be located in areas with constant and sufficiently strong winds to ensure efficient operation.

Wind turbine design and installation must take into account factors such as wind speed, distance from homes and environmental impact. Maintenance includes regular inspection of blades and mechanical components to ensure optimal operation and extend the life of the plant.

The installation of wind turbines requires a site assessment to determine the speed and consistency of the wind. Turbines must be mounted on suitable towers to obtain the necessary height to capture stronger and more constant winds. The position of turbines must be carefully chosen to avoid interference with buildings or other structures and to ensure safety during installation and operation.

For wind turbines, maintenance includes regular inspection of blades, mechanical components and control systems. The blades should be inspected for damage or ice build-up and the rotating mechanisms should be lubricated and adjusted to ensure smooth operation. It is important to monitor the system for abnormal vibrations or noise that could indicate problems.

**Wind Generator**

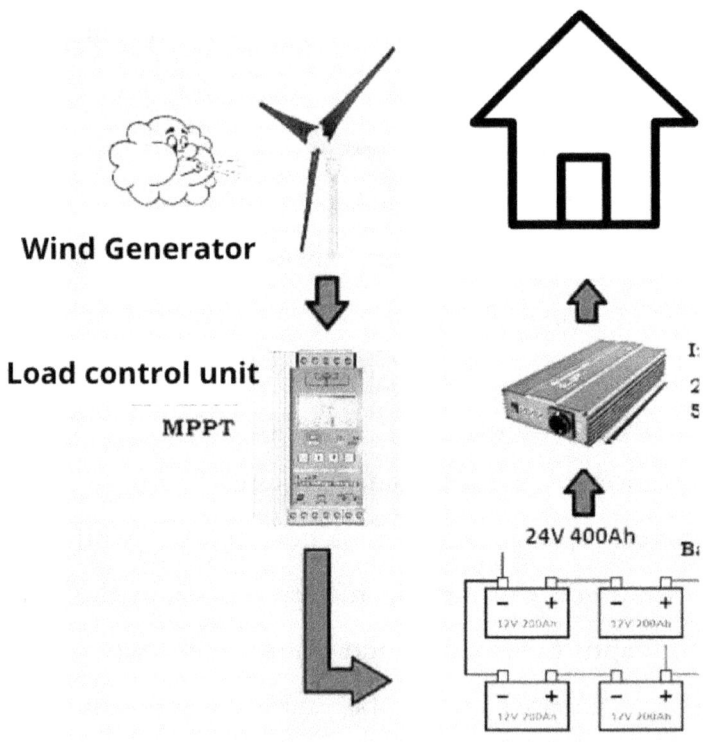

## Hydroelectric

L'energia idroelettrica sfrutta il movimento dell'acqua per generare elettricità. Questa fonte di energia può essere ottenuta attraverso grandi dighe che accumulano acqua e rilasciano flussi controllati per far girare le turbine, oppure attraverso impianti più piccoli come quelli micro-idroelettrici che utilizzano flussi d'acqua più modesti.

Le centrali idroelettriche tradizionali richiedono la costruzione di grandi dighe, il che può comportare impatti ambientali significativi e cambiamenti nei corsi d'acqua. Tuttavia, i sistemi micro-idroelettrici, che non richiedono grandi sbarramenti, offrono una soluzione più ecologica e sostenibile per le aree con corsi d'acqua naturali.

L'energia idroelettrica è molto affidabile e può fornire una fonte continua di energia se gestita correttamente. Tuttavia, è importante monitorare e gestire gli impatti ambientali e le modifiche ai flussi d'acqua per preservare gli ecosistemi circostanti e garantire la sostenibilità a lungo termine.

## Installazione di sistemi energetici

L'installazione di sistemi di energia rinnovabile richiede un'attenta pianificazione e competenze specialistiche per garantire che i sistemi funzionino in modo efficace e sicuro. La fase di installazione inizia con una valutazione delle condizioni locali, compresa l'analisi delle risorse energetiche disponibili quali radiazione solare, velocità del vento e flusso d'acqua.

## Micro-Hydro Systems

For micro-hydraulic systems, it is essential to analyze the flow and flow of water. These systems are often installed in natural watercourses and require the construction of canals or pipes to transport water to the turbines. It is important to ensure that the installation does not significantly alter the river ecosystem and that the system is integrated sustainably.

Maintenance of micro-hydro systems involves the regular cleaning of turbines and filters to ensure optimal water flow and prevent debris accumulation. Monitoring water quality and system performance is essential to ensure that the energy produced remains constant and that the plant operates efficiently.

Efficient management and regular maintenance of renewable energy systems not only ensure the sustainability and reliability of energy sources but also extend the useful life of plants, Contributing to efficient and sustainable energy management.

## Energy management and maintenance

The operation and maintenance of renewable energy systems is essential to ensure continuous and reliable operation. Energy management includes consumption planning and storage management, where applicable, to optimize the use of available resources and ensure a constant supply of energy.

# CHAPTER 6.

## EMERGENCY PREPAREDNESS

### First aid

First aid is essential in any emergency and can make the difference between rapid recovery and serious complications. It includes a series of techniques and procedures to stabilize an injured or ill person until professional medical help arrives. First aid skills include the ability to perform cardiopulmonary resuscitation (CPR), treat wounds and burns, and manage emergencies such as choking and shock.

The first step in any emergency room is to assess the safety of the scene to prevent further damage. It is important to assess the victim's condition and provide appropriate assistance, such as chest compressions and artificial respiration in case of cardiac arrest or airway decomposition in case of suffocation. First aid may also include managing bleeding, treating fractures, and administering emergency drugs such as adrenaline for severe allergic reactions.

First aid training is essential for everyone, not just professional rescuers. First aid courses, often offered by organizations such as the Red Cross, provide the practical and theoretical skills needed to deal effectively with emergencies. It is important to regularly update these skills and practice techniques to keep you on alert when needed

## Treatment of common wounds

Treating common wounds requires specific knowledge and practical skills to ensure optimal healing and prevent complications. The most common injuries are cuts, abrasions, bruises, and contusions. The first stage of treatment is complete cleaning of the wound to prevent infection. Using clean water and soap to gently wash the wound, followed by applying a disinfectant such as povidone-iodine or alcohol, helps eliminate bacteria and other impurities.

For deeper wounds or bleeding, apply direct pressure with sterile gauze to control the bleeding. In the case of more serious injuries, such as those with foreign bodies or tears, it is essential to seek professional medical assistance. Bruises, which are bruises caused by trauma, can be treated with cold packs to reduce swelling and relieve pain.

Burns should be treated with care. Immediately remove the heat source and cool the burned area with cold water for at least 10 minutes. Apply a sterile non-adhesive dressing and do not use ice or butter, as these can make the situation worse. Monitor burns for signs of infection and seek medical attention if the injury is extensive or severe.

## Preparazione di un kit di pronto soccorso

Preparing a complete first aid kit is essential to deal with emergency situations effectively. A well-equipped kit can make the difference between timely handling and worse. The kit must be easily accessible and contain a variety of supplies and equipment to deal with the most common emergencies.

A basic first aid kit should include sterile bandages of different sizes, gauze pads, patches, tweezers, scissors, and a thermometer. It is important to include disinfectants such as alcohol and povidone, as well as an antibiotic ointment to prevent infection. You may also want to add a pair of disposable gloves, a CPR mask and a flashlight with spare batteries.

In addition, the kit must contain basic drugs such as analgesics (ibuprofen or paracetamol), antihistamines and an oral rehydrating solution to treat dehydration. It is also advisable to include a first aid manual or emergency guide to provide detailed instructions on treatments.

The first aid kit must be checked and replenished regularly. Checking the expiry dates of medicines and replacing used or damaged supplies ensures that the kit is always ready for use in case of an emergency.

Basic supplies

Bandages and gauze

Elastic bandages of various sizes

Sterile gauze (in various sizes)

Medical tape

Patches of different sizes and shapes

Triangular band (for bandages or support)

**First aid equipment**

Rounded-tip scissors (for cutting bandages or clothes)

Tweezers (to remove splinters or spines)

Digital thermometer

Safety pins (for securing bandages or bandages)

Nitrile gloves (for protection against contamination)

Sterile cotton swabs

Cotton applicators (cotton-tipped)

Bags of instant ice

**Wound Treatment**

Antiseptic wipes

Disinfectant (for example, saline, iodine, or hydrogen peroxide)

Antibiotic ointment (like Neosporin)

Steri-strip (to close small wounds or cuts)

**Waterproof dressings**

Blister patches

Basic medicinal products

Analgesics (e.g., ibuprofen, paracetamol)

Antihistamines (for allergic reactions)

Antidiarrheal (such as loperamide)

Antinausea (like meclizine or ginger)

Sunburn ointment (for example, aloe vera cream)

Hydrocortisone cream (for itching or inflammation of the skin)

Burn dressing (as gel or impregnated bandages)

Activated carbon tablet (for poisoning)

**Resuscitation and Respiration**

Mask for CPR resuscitation

Isothermal blankets (space) to prevent hypothermia

**Support and Immobilization**

Folding splints (to immobilize fractures or sprains)

Elastic bandage (for support and compression)

**Specific treatment**

Kit for removing ticks

Snake bite kit (suction pump)

Ointment for insect bites

Lidocaine gel (for topical pain relief)

Sterile eye solution (for washing the eyes)

Oral antiseptic (for wounds or oral infections)

**Survival and Safety Materials**

Emergency whistle

Torch or headlamp with spare batteries

Fire-fighting or waterproof matches

Multi-purpose knife or folding blade

**Documentation**

First aid manual or information sheet

List of allergies and personal medical conditions

Copy of medical information and emergency contacts

**Other**

Sealable plastic bags (for safe disposal of biomedical waste)

Waterproof backpack or sturdy case to keep everything organized and dry

## Planning for natural disasters

Natural disaster planning is crucial to minimise risks and ensure an effective response in emergency situations. Natural disasters include events such as earthquakes, hurricanes, floods and forest fires, each of which requires specific preparation. Planning should start with an assessment of local risks and vulnerabilities, taking into account the geographical and climatic characteristics of the area.

It is essential to create a family emergency plan. This plan should include evacuation routes, meeting points and emergency contacts. Ensuring that all family members know the plan and actions to take in the event of a disaster is crucial. In addition, preparing an emergency kit with food, water, medicines and basic necessities for at least 72 hours is a prudent measure.

It is also important to know the resources and responses of local authorities, such as evacuation plans and available shelters. Participation in exercises and preparation courses can improve real-world emergency response capacity and preparedness. Monitoring the weather forecast and maintaining an open channel of communication with local authorities helps to receive timely updates and follow the evacuation or shelter.

## Evacuation strategies

Evacuation strategies are essential to ensure safe and rapid exit from risk areas during an emergency. Effective evacuation planning includes the definition of safe routes, preparation of a transport plan and communication with all family or group members.

Start with an assessment of the available evacuation routes and choose the safest and fastest ways out of the danger zone. It is essential to take account of traffic conditions and possible road closures. The supply of alternatives should be blocked or impracticable.

Prepare a transport plan that considers both own and public transport. Make sure the vehicle is in good condition, with a full tank and emergency kit on board. If you rely on public transport, knowing the times and stops of emergency lines can be useful.

Communicating the evacuation plan to all family members and neighbors, if possible, is essential. Establishing a safe meeting point and making sure everyone knows where to go in the event of separation is an important measure. During evacuation, maintaining calm and following the instructions of authorities is essential to ensure safety and reduce the risk of accidents.

# Essential concepts for an evacuation plan

## 1. Risk assessment

- Threat Identification: Assess the specific risks for your area, such as earthquakes, hurricanes, floods or forest fires.
- Vulnerability Analysis: Identifies vulnerable people (children, the elderly, people with disabilities) and considers special needs.
- Escape Route Planning: Identify and map out the main and alternative escape routes from home, work or school.

## 2. Creation of the Evacuation Plan

- Role Assignment: Assign specific responsibilities to each family or group member, such as who collects the emergency kit, who checks that everyone is evacuated, and who takes care of children or pets.
- Meeting Point: Establish a safe and well-known meeting point for everyone, both inside and outside your community. For example, a local park or a relative's house outside the danger zone.
- Evacuation Routes: Plan multiple evacuation routes, avoiding hazardous areas. Consider alternative means of transport, such as walking or cycling if the roads are blocked.

## 3. Communication

- Emergency Contacts: Compile a list of emergency phone numbers and emergency contacts, including family members, friends, and local emergency agencies.
- Communication Plan: Define a method for staying in touch during the evacuation, such as using mobile phones, walkie-talkies or a messaging app.
- Alert System: Subscribe to local alert systems to receive early warnings of imminent hazards.

## 4. Preparation of the Emergency Kit

- Essential Contents: Prepare a kit with water, non-perishable food, medicines, important documents, first aid kits, torches, batteries, local maps, and cash.
- Ease of Transport: Use a sturdy backpack or a wheeled bag to facilitate transportation.
- Duplicate Kits: If possible, prepare multiple kits and keep them in different places, such as at home, in the car, or at work.

## 5. Training and Simulations

- Evacuation Drills: Perform regular drills with all members of the group, practicing different emergency situations and checking the effectiveness of escape routes and meeting points.
- Plan Review: Review and update the evacuation plan periodically, especially after an exercise or if circumstances change (for example, if you move into a new home).

## 6. Evacuation in Emergency

- Act Quickly: Follow the evacuation plan immediately when you receive a warning or if the danger is obvious.
- Check and Report: Before leaving the area, make sure everyone is present and report your location to a designated emergency contact.
- Watch for updates: While evacuee, pay attention to updates via radio, social media, or local alert systems to know the situation and adapt the route if necessary.

## 7. Post-Emergence

- Safe Return: Return to the affected area only when local authorities confirm that it is safe to do so.
- Support and Recovery: Seek assistance for any reconstruction or psychological needs, and update the evacuation plan to prevent future emergencies.

## Temporary shelters

Temporary shelters provide additional protection and security during and after an emergency. These shelters can range from tents and mobile homes to more permanent structures such as prefabricated housing modules. The choice of temporary shelter depends on the nature of the emergency and the resources available.

For short-term emergencies, such as extreme weather events, tents can offer a quick and flexible solution. Tents should be installed in safe, dry areas away from potential hazards such as unstable trees or flooded areas. It is important to make sure that the tents are well anchored and equipped with drainage systems to prevent water infiltration.

For long-term emergencies, such as floods or fires, mobile homes or prefabricated modules can provide additional protection and comfort. These facilities must be located in safe areas and equipped with essential supplies such as water, food and sanitation. Maintenance and operation of temporary shelters shall include regular supervision to ensure that conditions remain safe and hygienic.

The preparation of temporary shelters should also take into account the availability of resources and health care. Establishing a plan for the distribution of essential goods and services is important to ensure the well-being of occupants and facilitate post-emergency recovery.

## Disaster response programme

In the event of natural disasters, it requires a systematic and well-organized approach to ensure the safety and security of all those involved. Here is a well-defined program with actions to be carried out systematically:

### 1. Risk Assessment

- Identify Potential Disasters: Analyze the region to determine which natural disasters are most likely (earthquakes, floods, hurricanes, fires, etc.).
- Assess Vulnerability: Examine structures, infrastructure and population to understand which are most vulnerable to these events.
- Risk Mapping: Create detailed maps of the most at-risk areas, indicating safe and avoid zones.

### 2. Development of the Emergency Plan

- Creating a Crisis Team: Form a team responsible for emergency management, with clear roles and specific responsibilities.
- Establish Evacuation Procedures: Define safe evacuation routes, collection points, and temporary shelters.
- Emergency Communication: Prepare a communication plan to keep everyone informed during and after the event,

including emergency numbers, radio channels, and social media.
- Contingency Plan for Essential Services: Organize strategies to quickly maintain or restore access to food, water, energy, and medical care.

## 3. Preparation and Training
- Personnel Training: Provides training for the crisis team and employees on emergency equipment use and evacuation procedures.
- Simulations and Exercises: Schedule periodic simulations to test the effectiveness of the emergency plan and make improvements.
- Emergency Kit: Assign or make available an emergency kit for each individual, containing food, water, medicines, first aid tools, torches, batteries, etc.

## 4. Community involvement
Education and Awareness: Organize workshops and distribute educational materials to the community to prepare them for possible disasters.

Collaboration with local authorities: Work closely with local governments, law enforcement, and emergency services to ensure effective coordination.

Creating Support Networks: It fosters neighborhood networks and mutual help groups to support the most vulnerable, such as elderly people and people with disabilities.

## 5. Monitoring and updating of the plan
- Continuous Monitoring: Use monitoring and early warning tools to identify early signs of an impending disaster.
- Periodic Review: Review the contingency plan at least once a year to update it based on new information or changes in circumstances.
- Documentation: Keep accurate records of all stages of planning, resources used, and lessons learned during the exercises.

## 6. Emergency response
- Plan Activation: As soon as an imminent risk is identified, activate the emergency plan, alerting the crisis team and the population.
- Evacuation and Security: Perform evacuation procedures, ensuring that everyone reaches the safe areas.
- Communications Management: Maintain constant communication to update the population on the evolution of the situation.

## 7. Recovery and Reconstruction

- Damage Assessment: After the disaster, assess the material damage and impact on the population.
- Victim Support: Provide immediate assistance to the injured and displaced, offering food, shelter, and psychological support.
- Reconstruction Plan: Create and implement a reconstruction plan to restore damaged infrastructure and improve resilience against future disasters.

## 8. Review and Improvement

- Lessons Learned: After the emergency, conduct a thorough review of actions taken to identify what worked and what can be improved.
- Plan Update: Integrate lessons learned into the emergency plan to improve response to future disasters.

# CHAPTER 7.

## SURVIVAL SKILLS

### Light the fire

Lighting a fire is one of the fundamental skills for survival and can be achieved through traditional and modern methods. Fire not only provides heat and light but is essential for cooking food, sterilizing water, and protecting wildlife.

### Traditional and modern methods

Traditional methods for starting fire include the use of steel and flint, wood friction, and the method of firing fire. The flint and flint method consists of striking the flint against the flint to produce sparks that ignite a combustible material such as cotton or steel wool. The wood friction method involves the use of a stick and a wooden board to generate heat through friction until a glowing charcoal is produced. The fire percussion method uses a piece of iron and an iron or obsidian stone to generate sparks.

Among modern methods, the most common are matches and lighters. Matches can be safety or phosphorous type and are generally easy to use, lighters can be gas or petrol and are very practical for starting a fire quickly.

**Fuel storage**

Fuel conservation is crucial to ensure the availability of resources in an emergency. Fuel, such as wood, coal, and synthetic materials, should be stored in a dry and well-ventilated place to avoid moisture and decomposition. For wood, it is advisable to stack so that the air can circulate freely around the logs. Using airtight containers for fuels such as coal and torches can extend their life and maintain their efficiency.

**Navigation and orientation**
**Using compasses and maps**

Navigation and orientation are key skills for survival in the open. The compass and maps are essential tools to determine one's own position and plot the route to a destination. The compass, which measures direction based on the Earth's magnetic fields, is a precise instrument that helps to maintain a correct course. It is important to understand how to read and interpret the cardinal points and how to align the compass with a map to plan the route.

Topographic maps provide details of terrain features, such as hills, valleys, and watercourses, and help identify landmarks. It is essential to be able to orient the map correctly and use the compass to trace the route and avoid getting lost.

## Natural navigation techniques

Natural navigation techniques are based on observation of the surrounding environment. Explorers can orient themselves using the sun, stars, and terrain. For example, the sun rises in the east and sets in the west, providing a general indication of directions. The position of stars, such as the Ursa Major, can be used to find the North at night. Land features such as water courses which generally run downstream can guide navigation without the aid of technological tools

## Craft techniques
### Wood and stone processing

Woodworking and stone is a vital survival skill that allows you to create tools, repairs, and other useful items. The woodworking can start with choosing the appropriate wood type, depending on the intended use. Hardwood, such as oak, is ideal for heavy instruments, while softwood, such as pine, is easier to work with. The main tools are knives, axes, and saws. The processing involves cutting, sanding, and shaping of wood to obtain functional shapes and tools.

Stoneworking requires tools such as hammers and chisels to sculpt and shape the stone. Stone can be used to build durable structures, such as walls and stoves, or to create tools like millstones and arrowheads. The choice of stone type is important; some stones, such as obsidian, can be easily chipped to create sharp edges.

## Manufacture of tools and weapons

Making tools and weapons is an essential part of survival and may include creating items such as knives, spears, and axes. Tools are essential for everyday activities such as cutting, digging, and building, while weapons can be used for defense and hunting. Production begins with the choice of materials, which can range from metals and wood to stones and bones. Manufacturing methods include forging, casting, and chipping to achieve desired shapes and functionality.

### 1. Lance

The spear is one of the oldest and most versatile weapons for hunting and defense.

Materials required:

A long, straight stick (about 1.5-2 meters)

A sharp stone, a sharp piece of metal, or a knife

Rope, twine, or lianas

Instructions for construction:

Preparation of the Stick: Find a sturdy stick, preferably made of hardwood such as ash or oak. Remove the bark and smooth the stick.

Tip of the spear: Sharpen one end of the stick until it is sharp.

If you have a sharp knife or stone, attach it to the end of the stick using a cord or twine.

Strengthening: To make the tip more resistant, you can harden it by cooking it on the fire for a few minutes. This process dries the wood and makes it harder.

Blade Attachment (optional): If you are using a sharp blade or stone, make sure it is firmly attached to the tip of the spear.

Use:

The spear can be used both for hunting small animals and for self-defense against predators.

## 2. Bow and Arrow

The bow is one of the most effective weapons for hunting, allowing to hit targets at a distance.

Materials required:

A long, flexible branch (wood like yew, elm or ash)

Sturdy twine or animal tendon

Straight sticks for arrows

Sharp stones or metal pieces for arrowheads

Feathers (optional)

Instructions for construction:

Construction of the Arch:

Choose a branch that is about 1.2-1.5 meters long. Make sure it is flexible but durable.

Cut a notch on both ends of the branch to secure the rope.

Secure the twine in the notches, creating adequate tension.

The Arrows' Realization:

Find straight sticks about 60-70 cm long.

Sharpen one end of the stick or add a stone or metal tip.

Attach feathers to the base of arrows to stabilize them in flight (if available).

Use:

The bow and arrows are great for hunting medium-sized game and can also be used for distance defense.

## 3. Slingshot

The slingshot is a simple but effective weapon for hitting small targets at medium range.

Materials required:

Elastic rubber strips (you can also use bicycle air chambers)

A piece of sturdy leather or fabric for the bag

A Y-shaped stick

Instructions for construction:

Preparation of the Frame: Find a sturdy Y-shaped stick. Smooth any roughness.

Fixing the Rubber: Attach a strip of rubber to each of the top ends of the Y. Make sure it is securely fastened.

Construction of the Bag: Attach the piece of leather or fabric to the center of the rubber strips to form the bag that will hold the bullets.

Use:

The sling can be used to hunt small animals such as birds or rabbits. It is also useful for self-defense at short range.

Use:

The sling can be used to hunt small animals such as birds or rabbits. It is also useful for self-defense at short range.

## 4. Snare Trap

Although not a traditional weapon, a snare trap is essential for survival, allowing you to catch animals without having to actively hunt them.

Materials required:

Strong wire, rope, or vines

Flexible branches for trap mechanism

Instructions for construction:

Preparation of the Lace: Create a sliding ring with the wire or rope.

Plant the Trap: Attach the ring to a flexible branch or solid base. The trap should be placed along the paths of the animals so that the ring is tightened around their head or paws when they pass.

## Creation of clothing and accessories

Creating clothes and accessories is an important skill for survival, as it provides protection and comfort in harsh environments. The processing of materials for clothing includes the processing of leather, natural fabrics, and plant fibers. Leather can be tanned and sewn to make jackets, boots, and other durable items. Natural fabrics, such as cotton and wool, can be worked by hand or with rudimentary tools to produce warm, breathable clothes.

The creation of accessories such as hats, gloves, and belts can further improve protection and efficiency. The use of natural dyeing and decoration techniques can add functionality and aesthetics to garments, improving their resistance to environmental conditions and user comfort.

Creating clothing and accessories for survival in nature requires ingenuity and the use of natural or recycled materials available in the surrounding environment. Here are some ideas for making headbands, belts, bandages, clothes, shoes, and other accessories useful in survival situations.

### 1. Bands

The bands are versatile and can be used to cover the head, retain sweat or even as improvised bandages.
Materials:
Fabric strips (may come from damaged clothes or blankets)
Internal bark of trees such as lime or willow

Broad and strong leaves, like those of the palm

Instructions:
- Fabric: Cut long, narrow strips of fabric from a t-shirt, pants or blanket. Tie the ends together to form a sash.
- Bark: Carefully remove the outer bark of a tree and collect the inner bark. Let the bark dry slightly and weave strips to create a durable band.
- Leaves: Weave strong, wide leaves, making sure you secure the ends.

## 2. Belts

Belts are essential for keeping your pants in place, carrying tools or even as laces for traps.

Materials:
- Natural ropes (e.g. lianas or vegetable fibres)
- Strips of leather (from hunted animals)
- Strips of sturdy fabric

Instructions:
- Ropes: Weave natural ropes to create a sturdy belt. You can add a hook or knot to tie it.
- Skin: If you have access to an animal's skin, cut a long and wide strip. Soften the skin by rubbing it and folding it repeatedly.
- Fabric: Cut a long, sturdy strip from a jacket or trousers and sew or knot the ends.

## 3. Clothes

Creating clothes in nature takes a little creativity, but it's possible with the right materials.

Materials:
- Animal skin
- Large and strong leaves
- Vegetable fibres

Instructions:
- Animal Skin: If you can hunt an animal, you can use the skin to make clothes. After you have treated and softened the skin, you can sew together pieces of leather using tendons or natural cords.
- Leaves: Weave broad, strong leaves together to create a kind of tunic or skirt. Use plant fibers to tie the leaves together.
- Plant Fibers: Collect and weave plant fibers such as hemp or jute to create basic clothing. This method takes time and patience but can result in durable clothing.

## 4. Shoes

Shoes are essential to protect your feet from difficult terrain.

Materials:
- Animal skin
- Tree bark
- Vegetable fibres

Instructions:
- Animal Skin: After softening the skin, cut it into the shape

of your feet with a little margin to sew the side parts. Use tendons or cords to sew the sides and add a shoelace to tighten the shoe around the ankle.
- Bark: Collect and work the bark of a tree as resistant as birch. Model it around the foot and secure it with lianas or natural ropes. This type of footwear is less durable but useful in case of emergency.
- Plant Fibers: Weave the fibers together to create a sandal or sole. You can then tie the sole to your foot with additional fibers or strips of leather.

## 5. Backpacks and bags

Backpacks and bags are useful for carrying supplies and equipment.

Materials:
- Animal skin
- Robust fabric
- Vegetable fibres

Instructions:
- Animal Skin: Cut a large piece of leather and sew the edges to create a bag or backpack. Add straps using leather cords or strips.
- Fabric: Use sturdy fabric to create a shoulder bag. Sew the ends and create a carrying strap.
- Plant Fibres: Weave the plant fibers to create a net or bag. This method takes time but can result in a resistant container.

# CHAPTER 8.

## LIVING IN HARMONY WITH NATURE

Principles of environmental sustainability

Living in harmony with nature requires a conscious commitment to environmental sustainability. This principle implies the adoption of practices that reduce the negative impact of human activities on the environment and promote ecological balance. Waste reduction through recycling and re-use is crucial. For example, avoiding the use of single-use plastics and opting for biodegradable or recyclable materials significantly contributes to reducing pollution.

Energy efficiency is another pillar of sustainability. The use of renewable energy sources, such as solar and wind, reduces dependence on fossil fuels and greenhouse gas emissions. In addition, the design of green buildings that maximize the use of natural light and improve thermal insulation can reduce energy consumption.

Sustainable management of soil and water resources is essential to preserve ecosystems. Agricultural practices, such as crop rotation and cultivation of local plants, can maintain soil fertility and prevent erosion. In addition, the conscious use of water, through techniques such as drip irrigation and rainwater harvesting, helps to maintain water balance and reduce resource scarcity.

## Conservation of natural resources

Conserving natural resources is crucial to ensuring that the planet's resources remain available for future generations. This practice includes protecting natural habitats, reducing excessive consumption, and adopting sustainable production methods. Protecting wilderness areas and nature reserves helps to preserve biodiversity and ecosystems vital for life on Earth.

Reducing the waste of resources through the adoption of responsible consumption habits is another important strategy. This may include choosing local and seasonal products, that reduce transport-related carbon emissions, and supporting producers who adopt green practices. Furthermore, the implementation of waste recovery and treatment technologies can help reduce pressure on landfills and improve the quality of the environment.

## Education and Knowledge Sharing

Educating and sharing knowledge about environmental sustainability is essential to promote a culture of respect and care for nature. Educational programs in schools and communities can raise awareness of sustainability principles and everyday practices that reduce environmental impact. The creation of practical workshops and awareness-raising activities, such as sustainable gardening or waste management workshops, helps to pass on useful skills and encourage eco-friendly behavior.

Knowledge sharing can also take place through networks of communities and interest groups promoting green practices. Initiatives such as time banks, where people exchange services and skills related to sustainability, can strengthen social cohesion and promote the adoption of sustainable lifestyles.

Digital media and platforms play a crucial role in disseminating information. Blogs, podcasts, and social media can be effective tools to educate a wider audience and stimulate debate on environmental issues. Creating informative and engaging content helps to reach different segments of the population and encourages the adoption of eco-sustainable behavior at a global level.

# Conclusion

## Key Points Summary

In conclusion, off-grid life represents a deeply conscious and self-sufficient approach to live in harmony with nature and reduce dependence on modern infrastructure. We explored various aspects essential for living off-grid, starting from water management and food sustainability, to the construction of shelters and the use of renewable energy.

In the chapter on water management, we saw how crucial it is to identify and exploit reliable and sustainable water sources, such as rainwater harvesting and well-building. Water purification, through methods such as filtration and chemical treatment, ensures the safety and health of the water consumed.

Food sustainability has been addressed with attention to food production methods such as permaculture and small-space gardening. Diversification of food supply sources, including hunting, fishing and gathering wild plants, is essential to ensure a balanced diet. Furthermore, food preservation techniques such as canning and dewatering are essential for efficient management of food resources.

Shelter construction was analyzed in terms of planning, choice of materials and construction techniques. We discussed how natural materials such as earth, wood and stone can be used to create safe and durable structures, emphasizing the importance of insulation and energy efficiency.

In the renewable energy chapter, the various available energy systems were explored, including solar, wind and hydro. The correct installation and maintenance of these systems is crucial to ensure a stable and sustainable energy supply.

We covered emergency preparedness, first aid, preparation of emergency kits and evacuation strategies. These skills are essential to deal with unforeseen situations with confidence and readiness.

**Inspiration for off-grid life**

Living off-grid is a path that requires dedication and preparation, but offers a life full of freedom and connection with nature. Embracing this way of life means adopting a sustainability-oriented mindset The European Commission has published a report on the EU's energy research and development program.

Every aspect of off-grid life, from resource management to the construction and maintenance of energy plants, contributes to a harmonious and sustainable living environment. Embracing these practices can also be an inspiration, demonstrating how simplicity and efficiency can lead to a more fulfilling life in balance with the environment.

The choice to live off-grid can also promote a renewed respect for nature and a greater awareness of one's own resources and needs. Every step towards self-sufficiency is a step towards a more conscious and rewarding life, in which daily challenges are faced with resilience and creativity.

**Resources and suppliers**

To live off-grid effectively, it is essential to know the resources and suppliers that can provide the necessary materials and tools. This section provides a list of reliable sources for equipment and materials purchase, as well as educational resources for further in-depth research.

Renewable energy suppliers: Companies offering solar panels, wind turbines and hydroelectric systems. It is useful to consult their websites for product information, installation options, and maintenance.

Building material suppliers: shops and companies selling materials for the construction of shelters, such as wood, stone, and insulation materials. Some may also offer consultancy services to design and build effective shelters.

Educational resources: books, online courses, and workshops dedicated to off-grid life, permaculture, and environmental sustainability. These resources provide practical and theoretical knowledge essential for managing a self-sufficient life.

## Glossary of technical terms

- Ignition of the Fire: The act of creating and maintaining a flame using different methods, such as steel and flint, matches, lighters, or primitive techniques like the bow from fire.
- Acclimation: The process of adaptation of the human body to new environmental conditions, such as high altitudes or extreme temperatures.
- Aquaculture: Cultivation of aquatic organisms, such as fish, crustaceans, and algae, in controlled environments for consumption or other purposes.
- Adaptation: Ability to change behaviors, habits, and techniques in response to changes in the surrounding environment or available resources.
- Adobe: Bricks made of clay, sand, and straw, are used in the construction of structures for their thermal insulation capacity.
- Solar Alambic: A device that uses the heat of the sun to distill water, separating it from contaminants and making it drinkable.
- Red Alert: An emergency where an immediate response is required to protect life and property.
- Handicraft: Manual skills required to create tools, weapons, clothing, and other items using natural or recycled materials.

- Self-defense: Techniques and strategies used to protect against physical attacks or other threats.

- Compasses and Maps: Essential tools for navigating in unfamiliar environments, used to orient oneself and find safe routes.

- Bushcraft: The set of skills and knowledge to live and thrive in natural environments using resources available in nature.

- Hunting: The activity of chasing and capturing wild animals for food, using weapons, traps, or other techniques.

- Camping: The practice of staying temporarily outdoors, often used as a survival exercise.

- Truss: A triangular-shaped structure used in roofs to distribute weight and provide support.

- Water cycle: The continuous movement of water on Earth through evaporation, condensation, and precipitation, fundamental for the collection and conservation of water.

- Emergency food: Long-life foods, such as military rations, canned foods, and freeze-dried foods, which can be stored for emergencies.

- Natural Waterways: Streams, rivers, lakes, and other freshwater sources that can be used for water supply.

- Sensory deprivation: Reduction or absence of sensory stimuli, which can negatively affect survival abilities.

- Dehydration: The process of removing water from food to

prolong its storage or dangerous physical condition caused by lack of water intake.

- Distillation: Process of water purification by evaporation and subsequent condensation to remove impurities and contaminants.
- Emergency: An unforeseen and dangerous situation that requires immediate action to protect life, health, or property.
- Renewable Energy: Energy obtained from natural and sustainable sources, such as the sun, wind, and water, used to power devices and plants without exhausting non-renewable resources.
- Drying: A food preservation technique that involves the removal of water to prevent the growth of bacteria, mold, and yeast.
- Exposure: Dangerous condition of being subject to adverse weather conditions, such as cold, heat or rain, without adequate protection.
- Evacuation: The process of leaving a hazardous area in an organized and safe manner due to an impending or ongoing disaster.
- Fermentation: A chemical process in which sugars are transformed into alcohol, gas or acids by bacteria, yeasts or other microorganisms, used to preserve food.
- Water Filter: A device or method used to remove impurities,

particles and pathogens from the water to make it drinkable.
- Signal Fire: A fire lit in a specific way to attract the attention of rescuers or other survivors, often used in emergencies.
- Gardening: Growing plants for food, pleasure or beauty, which can be adapted to small spaces or for the production of food in survival situations.
- Urban gardening: Growing plants and vegetables in limited spaces such as balconies, roofs or small courtyards in the city.
- First Aid Kit: Collection of medical supplies and tools to treat wounds, diseases and other health emergencies.
- Woodworking: Ability to cut, shape, and work wood to create tools, shelters and other items necessary for survival.
- Natural navigation: Techniques of orientation based on natural signals such as the sun, stars, terrain formations and vegetation.
- Orientation: The act of determining one's own position and direction using maps, compasses or natural signals.
- Permaculture: A sustainable agricultural design system that mimics natural ecosystems to create a self-sustaining and sustainable environment.
- Fishing: Activity of catching fish from bodies of water for consumption, using baits, nets or other tools.
- Medicinal plants: Plants used to treat diseases and ailments, a

crucial resource in survival.

- Wild Edible Plants: Plants that grow naturally in nature and can be harvested and used as food.
- Well: Structure dug to access underground aquifers, providing drinking water.
- Emergency Preparedness: The process of planning and organizing resources, skills, and strategies to deal with crisis or disaster situations.
- Shelter project: Detailed planning of the construction of a shelter, including materials, design, and construction techniques.
- Proximity to water: Strategic choice of the location of a camp or shelter near a source of water to ensure continuous access to drinking water.
- Rainwater Collection: Technique of collecting and storing rainwater for domestic, agricultural, or emergency use.
- Rationing: Controlled and limited distribution of resources, such as food and water, to ensure long-term survival in situations of scarcity.
- Resilience: Ability to adapt and recover quickly from difficulties or changes, essential for long-term survival.
- Temporary Shelters: Improvised structures built with materials available on site to provide immediate protection from the weather.

- Local Resources: Materials and resources available in the surrounding environment, used to build shelters, make fire, and create tools.
- Sustainability: Practice of using resources in a way that does not deplete them, preserving the environment for future generations.
- Evacuation Strategies: Detailed plans for evacuating a hazardous area in a safe and organized manner.
- Hunting Techniques: Methods and tools used to locate, capture and kill wild animals for food.
- Conservation Techniques: Methods to preserve food and other resources to prolong their life span and prevent deterioration.
- Traps: Devices designed to capture wild animals without the need for direct contact.
- Ventilation: Systems or methods to ensure a constant flow of air within a shelter, preventing the accumulation of moisture and keeping the air fresh.
- Wilderness: Nature areas

www.ingramcontent.com/pod-product-compliance
Lightning Source LLC
Chambersburg PA
CBHW070827090825
30880CB00020B/352